Excelling in the Externship

Excelling in the Externship

A Preparation Guide for Medical Assisting and Allied Health

Kimberly Halverson-Bender,
M.S.

Prentice Hall
Upper Saddle River, New Jersey 07458

Library of Congress Cataloging-in-Publication Data

Halverson-Bender, Kimberly.
Excelling in the externship / Kimberly Halverson-Bender.—1st ed.
  p.cm.
Includes bibliographical reference.
ISBN-13: 978-0-13-501682-4
ISBN-10: 0-13-501682-7
1. Paramedical education.   I. Title
R847.H35 2010
610.73'7069—dc22   2008040039

Publisher: Julie Levin Alexander
Publisher's Assistant: Regina Bruno
Executive Editor: Joan Gill
Associate Editor: Bronwen Glowacki
Development Editor: Bronwen Glowacki
Director of Marketing: Karen Allman
Senior Marketing Manager: Harper Coles
Marketing Assistant: Crystal Gonzalez
Managing Production Editor: Patrick Walsh
Production Liaison: Julie Li
Production Editor: Tanushree Kanungo
Manufacturing Manager: Ilene Sanford
Manufacturing Buyer: Pat Brown
Senior Design Coordinator: Christopher Weigand
Cover Designer: Kevin Kall
Cover Image: New Vision Technologies Inc./Digital Vision/Getty Images
Composition: Aptara®, Inc.
Printing and Binding: Edwards Brothers
Cover Printer: Edwards Brothers

Pearson Education Ltd., London
Pearson Education Singapore, Pte. Ltd.
Pearson Education Canada, Inc.
Pearson Education—Japan
Pearson Education Australia Pty. Limited

Pearson Education North Asia, Ltd., Hong Kong
Pearson Educación de Mexico, S.A. de C.V.
Pearson Education Malaysia Pte. Ltd.
Pearson Education Upper Saddle River, New Jersey

Prentice Hall
is an imprint of

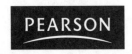

www.pearsonhighered.com

10 9 8
ISBN-13: 978-0-13-501682-4
ISBN-10:   0-13-501682-7

Contents

Chapter Three   Externship Interviews   27

Chapter Four   Attitudes and Perceptions   39

Chapter Five   Etiquette and Professional Manners 57

Chapter Six   Developing Professional Relationships 69

Chapter Seven   Fulfilling the Student Role During the Externship 81

Preface

The progression from completing the allied health program of study to becoming a professional within the industry is bridged by the externship. This externship is the time and place in which the student has the opportunity to begin building professional relationships and to show off his or her technical skills and unique talents in serving and working with others. It is a time when avoidable pitfalls should not interfere with various professional opportunities. To make the most of the externship, students must be well prepared to take on new challenges, act responsibly, learn proactively, and develop themselves professionally, which are all major goals of *Excelling in the Externship*.

The overall purpose of *Excelling in the Externship* is to present to students the full picture of the externship experience. Student readers will realize the value and purpose of the externship, will be prepared by being familiar with the expectations for all aspects of the journey, and will discover the benefits and opportunities that await them when they begin their careers with completion of a successful externship. They also will be given tips on the various pitfalls and mistakes to avoid in order to excel in the externship. Coverage of the externship from preterm to postterm is provided to guide students' focus and to help them maintain professionalism, responsibility, a positive attitude, and proactive learning throughout the process. The goal of this worktext is to prepare allied health externs for a successful practical experience. In turn, this helps student-graduates to launch their careers with confidence, motivation, and meaningful experience. This also helps educational institutions send well-prepared students who intend to succeed to their partnering or affiliated offices, hospitals, pharmacies, and other facilities.

The content covered in this text is based on a significant amount of experience I have had with students and their externships, which makes this worthwhile reading for any budding allied health professional approaching the externship phase. Many colleges and educational institutions may offer, or do not provide, very limited preparation for students in the specific, yet important, aspects of switching on the professionalism required in allied health fields, which actually must begin before or during the externship. This guide is intended to fill this gap in externship preparation when significant face-to-face time between instructors and students for this purpose is unachievable within the established curriculum. It can be used concurrently with other related course material or as an independent study for students prior to beginning an externship.

Excelling in the Externship is organized logically, beginning with introducing the purpose and value of the externship. The text then maps out what the externship site staff and the college or school expect of students. A chapter about externship interviews focuses on preparing students who are required to attend an interview prior to beginning the externship. Appropriate attitudes, etiquette, and the development of working professional relationships are discussed. Next, how students are to fulfill the student role through following instructions and engaging in proactive learning is explored. Meant to serve as motivation for students, the next section discusses the priceless benefits of completing an externship, some of which are tied to the specific training site. Material covering externship evaluations and grades touches on the conclusion of the externship phase. Real-life case studies follow. The final chapter explores the beginning of the job search for allied health careers.

Features of this text include the following:

- **Tips from Professionals.** Brief sections throughout this guide provide you with very up-front, practical advice from various industry professionals who have had ample experience working with and training student-externs. This is one of the most valuable features of this text. Based on their experiences with student-externs, theses individuals have kindly offered their foremost thoughts about preparing for the externship. Their specific thoughts have been contributed with the best interest of each student in mind. These insights from industry professionals support the many topics in this text while providing information and recommendations from real-life, experienced, externship site supervisors. So, consider the words of these experts carefully, as they will be reiterated throughout this guide because they are so relevant to externships.

- **Self-Prep Questions.** These questions are provided to guide and prepare students for each aspect of their externship experience. They prompt students to think about what they will do when put into certain situations, as well as how to evaluate and improve their performance. An example from Chapter 3 preps students by requiring them to think of questions to ask in an interview, while examples in Chapter 5 focus on aspects of their etiquette that they can improve. Students will find ample room to write their answers.

- **Role-Play Scenario.** Each chapter presents a role-playing scenario for students. Directions describe how to set up the scenario, and questions lead students to observe "what is wrong" and "what is right" about how everyone acts. Space for recording answers is provided.

- **Readiness Checklist.** All chapters conclude with a "Readiness Checklist" to ensure that students understand all the objectives presented within the chapter. Students will find a place to check off the objectives as they learn them.

- **Journal.** At the end of this book, lined pages are provided on which students can take notes as they make their way through the program or can journal their externship thoughts and experiences.

- **Folder.** The back cover of this book has a pocket in which students can keep any important papers or documents they might collect during their externship.

Acknowledgments

I would like to extend appreciation to the following reviewers for providing valuable feedback throughout the review process:

Dominica Austin, BSN
Academic Dean
Lincoln College of Technology
Marietta, Georgia

Tricia Berry, MATL, OTR/L
Director of Clinical Placement
Kaplan University

Beth Anne Buchholz, BS, CMA
Medical Assisting Department Chair
Wichita Area Technical College
Wichita, Kansas

Ursula Cole, MEd, CMA, CCS-P, CHI
Medical Program Coordinator
Indiana Business College

Dawn Eitel, AAS, CMA
Medical Assisting Program Director
Kirkwood Community College
Cedar Rapids, Iowa

Cindy Garman, CMA
Medical Program Director/Director of Career Services
Akron Institute
Akron, Ohio

Robyn Gohsman, AAS, RMA, CMAS
Medical Assisting Program Director
Medical Careers Institute
Newport News, Virginia

Lisa Nagle, BSEd, CMA
Medical Assisting Program Director
Augusta Technical Institute
Augusta, Georgia

Julie Rismiller, CMA
Clinical Externship Coordinator
Lincoln Technical Institute
Allentown, Pennsylvania

Janet Sesser, RMA, CMA, BS
Associate Vice President of Education
Chubb Institute
Phoenix, Arizona

Donna Stevenson, BA, LPN, CAHI
Allied Health Department Chair
Remington College
Largo, Florida

Nancy Wright, RN, BS CNOR
Instructor, School of Health Sciences
Virginia College
Birmingham, Alabama

Excelling in the Externship

Kimberly Halverson-Bender

chapter one

The Link Between Your Education and Your Career

Introduction

This chapter presents basic information concerning the logic behind the concept of the externship as an integral part of allied health career training. To add substance and reality to these introductory concepts, several factors to remember and practice are emphasized during this phase of learning. These considerations include gaining "real world" experience, functioning as part of an organized professional team, abiding by the major legal and ethical standards of the industry, and realizing the significance of applying professional skills such as organization, time management, and multitasking. The overall goal is to reveal how various topics and lessons from your classroom training will transfer into the real world in the externship. The chapter concludes with Self-Prep Questions, a Role-Play Scenario, and a Readiness Checklist.

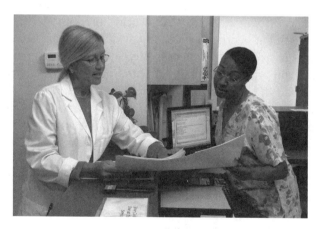

The externship provides students with valuable learning opportunities from professionals in the field of health care.

Chapter Objectives

- Identify the link from the classroom to the career created by the externship.
- Identify the basic meaning of *externship* and synonymous terms.
- Describe the overall purpose of the externship.
- Describe what it means to work as part of a health care team.
- Recall important legal and ethical considerations to be acted on during the externship.
- Describe how organizational and time management skills are important during the externship.
- Briefly describe *multitasking*.

The Importance of Your Externship

The time to prepare has arrived. You are likely in the final phases of your classroom training and are knocking on the door of your professional career in allied health. In addition to completing your classroom work, you need to take just one more step: the externship. Many students simply accept that they will fulfill an externship without actually understanding the reasons or priceless benefits of doing so. The reason is fairly simple: Practicing skills in the classroom is worlds apart from the "real world" medical office, clinic, outpatient surgery center, hospital, pharmacy, or other allied health setting.

The Big Transition: Student to Professional

Think of your externship as a bridge you must cross to go from the familiar, comfortable classroom to your "real world" professional career. In the classroom, a professional instructor is readily available to correct you and give you as many chances as you need to successfully acquire a certain skill or professional habit. Often, you are well acquainted with your classmates and instructors, and you are able and to learn within a happy comfort zone. This changes quite a bit the first day you step into your externship site. However, this shift from comfortable and familiar to uncomfortable and unfamiliar is for the best as it builds on your collection of professional experiences, and it is valuable to you personally in this way.

During the externship, it is understood by the office staff that you are an apprentice on the path to becoming an independent worker. While crossing the bridge, you have the experience of building your independence while simultaneously realizing your interdependence within a team, further developing your practical skills, and developing your professionalism in many other ways. Take advantage of the advice and constructive criticism offered to you by the professionals in this text; absorbing their insights will contribute greatly to your store of knowledge, and as you read you will become more aware of the many benefits of this phase of learning.

What Is Meant by Externship?

The word *externship* is interchangeable with the terms *practicum, practical experience, clinical rotation,* and *internship,* among others. All these terms directly capture the concept of students practicing clinical or other specialized practical skills in a professionally supervised, off-campus, real-world setting as part of a program of study. While an array of allied health specialties exists, each with its own unique set of required achievements for students in training, the common purpose of the externship experience among these allied health professions is to successfully apply relevant skills and knowledge in a professional setting. All clinically trained students must complete an externship, and even many administratively trained students are required to do so.

Applying Your Skills and Knowledge

Obviously, practicing your clinical and other practical skills is one of the most important objectives you will have to achieve. Some students think they will have the opportunity to acquire (rather than refine) their skills while practicing at the externship site. While some sites may provide time and an available staff member to assist trainees in mastering a certain skill, most office managers and facility supervisors expect that the student-extern has already mastered most necessary skills in the classroom portion of training. For example, reading a blood pressure is a skill that requires concentration, accuracy, and precision. It is a skill that must be learned through repetitious practice over time. It is expected that you are able to be productive in this particular skill if you are a medical assistant (MA); you should be comfortable with this task and effective when performing it since a busy facility allows no time to relearn skills practiced in the classroom.

The overall purpose of your externship, if clinically focused, is to apply the skills acquired in the classroom to a real-world setting where patients are sick, moody, depressed, agitated, or impatient with the prolonged process of checking in to see a physician. If your externship is, for example, in the realm of insurance and billing or health information, the general purpose will be to exercise your efficiency and accuracy in handling claims, using diagnosis and procedure codes, verifying insurance, discussing account information with patients and payers, functioning with the team, and so on, in a fast-paced setting where managers are concerned with timely and accurate reimbursement. For externships in pharmacy technology, students must focus on several areas, such as customer service, assisting in insurance verification, working within a team of one or more pharmacists and other technicians, and practicing proper handling and dispensing of drugs.

Professionalism: The Highest Calling

In all externships, utmost professionalism is expected of student-externs by all facility managers, doctors, pharmacists, and other health care professionals. Classroom time generally does not provide the opportunity to practice the more professional and personal side of working within the industry, and the externship experience is extremely valuable in polishing these skills. Various aspects of how one's level of professionalism affects an externship (and future career) are discussed throughout this text. For the benefit of all student readers, it is noted here that most externship failures or below-average outcomes are generally due to lack of professionalism. In other words, your effort to maintain your professionalism is usually the factor that determines the success or failure of your externship. Therefore, it is extremely important that you focus throughout your pre-externship classroom study on developing and refining your professional attributes for the sake of your externship and your soon-to-follow career.

Becoming Part of the Health Care Team

In medical assisting externships, in addition to helping to keep patients content and comfortable, you'll be practicing the art of participating as an active member of an important medical care team. This also entails developing skills that are unattainable solely from classroom experience. Today's medical office teams are expected to be efficient, but that efficiency must not compromise the effectiveness or quality of care provided to patients.

Typically, an average office staff might include the following:

- front desk personnel (covering reception, sign in, appointments, and handling faxes and phones)
- billing representatives
- patient records specialists
- an administrator or office manager
- specialized technicians (X-ray, phlebotomy, etc.)
- medical assistant(s)
- nurse(s)
- nurse practitioner(s) (ARNP)
- physician assistant(s) (PA)
- physician(s)

In particular, the MA is an important link between both front and back ends of the office. Likewise, those student-externs practicing in the specialty of administrative office, as well as billing and coding, must blend into a functioning team, effectively contributing to the tasks at hand so that the complete order and functioning of the facility are maintained. The team aspect is also a significant factor in the efficiency of pharmacies, dental offices, and so on. It is also important to practice the large-scale team concept that spans various facilities, recognizing the interdependency among all areas of patient service necessary for the overall delivery of health care. An example of this large-scale teamwork is the communication that takes place between the MA or nurse and the pharmacy technician when a prescription is ordered or called in for a patient.

The externship provides a golden opportunity to step into place as an integral part of this large-scale team, in whatever specialization you practice, proving to yourself and other professionals that you are a valuable asset. This type of learning experience is tremendously valuable and helps student-externs to develop professional skills that can be used in future career placement and advancement. The externship is likely to be the first place where education can be integrated as you practice in close association with other team members.

Gaining Experience with Legal and Ethical Considerations

Do you recall the medical law and ethics topics emphasized in your program of study? Do you remember the importance of professional liability issues, Health Information Portability and Accountability Act (HIPAA) compliance, patient confidentiality, the potential use of a patient's chart as a legal document, and such? Well, here it is, once again, in *real-world* application. Adhering to professional standards in these areas is extremely important. Directly applicable to your duties as an MA or other allied health professional, you will communicate constantly in-person (face-to-face), over the phone, via the fax, and probably through e-mail, primarily regarding patients and their ailments, health history, prescriptions, lab work and diagnostic testing, billing and insurance, office and facility issues, and so on. You must use professional discretion in how and where you communicate patient information to your co-workers. Basic behaviors you will need to practice are speaking softly and privately to your patients and customers, keeping medical charts closed when you are not making notes in them, and speaking softly over the phone if you are communicating with a patient or about a patient. Also, it is important to keep in mind the significance of every piece of information you record in a patient's file or chart; documentation must be accurate and correct because at any time any patient chart can be subpoenaed as a legal document for court proceedings. Unfortunately, substantial time is typically unavailable in the classroom setting for elaborate role-playing of these necessary applications. Practicing according to the applicable legal and ethical standards of your discipline is not only a requirement but also a critical component of your overall qualification to work successfully as an allied health professional.

Organization and Time Management Applications

Organization and time management are other professional skills you will build on during the externship. These are learned to some extent while attending class, managing your homework and projects, and studying for comprehensive exams. Perhaps you have had the opportunity to practice these in your previous employment endeavors. However, managing patients and helping maintain order in the office are, again, specific and necessary skills you can only learn by experience.

Chart or document organization, timeliness in preparing patient rooms, and efficiency in your clinical and administrative tasks are major areas in which you must demonstrate punctuality. Your performance should demonstrate quality work in which you perform at or above the professional standard of care and practice, not merely a haphazard effort to keep pace. Quality and correctness in your work apply as much as efficiency. You cannot afford to make mistakes when assessing vital signs, recording information in patient charts, or communicating information verbally to other medical office staff or to representatives in other facilities, while keeping in mind the legal aspects of the patient medical record.

Regardless of your area of practice, you will learn to multitask (i.e., to manage several different and possibly unrelated responsibilities in a given period of time). *Multitasking* is one of the buzzwords of today's workplace, and grasping how to implement it will build the list of professional skills you develop while on externship. Everyone working in your facility will have to manage their time, too. Learning how to effectively manage your time will provide you with another important, experience-based skill that you will need for a successful allied health career.

HIGHLIGHT: Tips from Professionals

"Students should take advantage of the externship opportunity and be professional, on time, and eager to help out. The value of the externship is based on the students' attitude and their open-mindedness. From my experience, students who learn the most are those who show the most enthusiasm and excitement. All my current employees were former externs at one point."

Advice and Recommendations

1. Be yourself. (This helps you to be more comfortable and have more confidence.)
2. Treat the externship as a job or a future job opportunity.
3. Have a positive attitude and show a willingness to learn.
4. Be on time. Call the externship site if you're running late or unable to get there.
5. Ask questions. It's okay if you're not sure of something or didn't learn something in school that you may work with at the site.

Louie Hilal
President and Owner of a Medical Billing Company

CONCLUSION

Many benefits and necessary considerations beyond those mentioned in this chapter are worth looking forward to, as you will learn in later chapters. However, this chapter addresses some of the foremost reasons why your externship is a necessary part of your comprehensive education and training as a medical assistant, health information technician, office assistant, pharmacy technician, dental hygienist, or other allied health professional. If this externship will be your first experience in any health care setting, the time you spend is even more valuable and important to you in your quest to enter the challenging yet rewarding industry of allied health.

Self-Prep Questions

1. What do you believe you personally have to gain from your externship?

   I think I will gain the confidence to work in a medical setting, learn how a real office operates, and skills and knowledge that cannot be learned in the classroom.

2. List at least five important purposes for completing the externship.

   ① To Graduate from school
   ② Gain experience and hands on skills
   ③ learn things that can't be learned in the classroom
   ④ Networking
   ⑤ Gaining references

3. Find out, write down, and remember the number of hours you are expected to complete. How many hours are required of you on a daily or weekly basis? If you are in a program with clinical rotations through different practice areas, write down your scheduled hour requirements for each rotation.

A total of 360 hours and a minimum of 30 a week.

4. What are three (at a minimum) basic skills you can practice to help ensure patient confidentiality?

① Don't discuss private pt info with anyone. ② Always lock computers. ③ Never leave papers laying out. ④ Keep files in appropriate places + covered. ⑤ Send faxes to secure fax machines. ⑥ Speak quietly with patients in waiting room and in front of others.

5. Why is accuracy of documentation in patient charts so important?

Patient records are legal documents and can be used as so in court cases. Also, it is important because the patients

total care and health is
maintained in the record and
based off of them.

Role-Play Scenario

Two individuals are needed for this scenario. Suppose it is your first day of externship. You walk into the medical office and tell the receptionist you are there to begin your externship and that you know you need to meet with Patty, the office manager, first. The receptionist locates Patty and informs her that you have arrived for your first day of externship. Role-play the scenario in which Patty comes to greet you, gives you an office overview and tour, and introduces you to the staff members. As Patty is talking with you and walking you through the office, demonstrate your overall idea of professionalism in this situation. To start, first consider some major aspects that contribute to professionalism.

1. How will you present yourself professionally to give a good first impression? Consider your dress and appearance, mannerisms, communication tactics, and so on.

I would be dressed as permitted to their
policies, hair and nails clean and groomed,
and firstly be on time. When greeting
I would shake hands, making eye contact
the whole time, saying it's nice to be
there. I would speak respectfully and
clearly to everyone, greet everyone in the
office. I would be very kind and curtious
to everyone, and offer my assistance
anywhere I could.

2. Since you do not know much about this office and how it functions yet, what are some intelligent questions you can ask Patty as she is introducing you to the office setting and staff? (Keep in mind that these types of questions demonstrate your overall interest in the profession and your desire to learn.)

①Ask how the office operates on a normal day.②How many physicians and other medical personel work on an average day.③Who to report any problems or issues to.④Who can I go to when I have any geestions.

Readiness Checklist

✓ I understand why the externship is required of health care professionals.

✓ I understand the differences between classroom learning and the experiential learning that I will complete during the externship.

✓ I understand what is meant by working as part of a professional team.

✓ I understand the importance of maintaining patient confidentiality and of measures such as HIPAA that ensure its maintenance.

✓ I know where I can find resources that will review the standard of care and code of ethics regarding my practice as a medical assistant or other health professional.

✓ I understand that I am to be discreet in communicating patient information.

✓ I understand the ways in which my organization, time management, and multitasking skills will be exercised during my externship.

chapter two

Meeting and Exceeding Expectations

Introduction

This chapter presents various expectations that all future externs should heed in advance of their externship. First, various common college, school, and departmental requirements are presented, followed by the expectations externship site

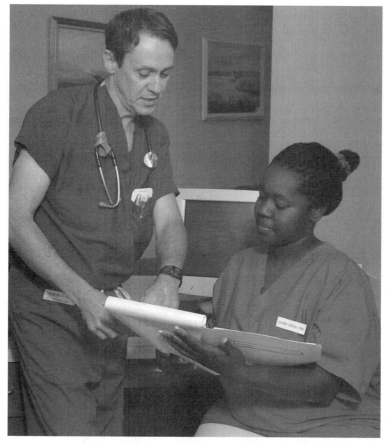

Externship site supervisors expect practicing students to take a proactive and professional approach in learning during the practicum.

managers and trainers have of externs. This foreknowledge will help you realize the importance of completing all documentation and other academic or college requirements on time, as well as understanding the minimum expectations held by the professionals providing your on-site training. The chapter concludes with Self-Prep Questions, a Role-Play Scenario, and a Readiness Checklist.

Chapter Objectives

- Identify the two parties to whom the student-extern is responsible.
- Recognize student-extern health documentation that may be required before externship.
- Identify the requirements typically imposed by career/professional services departments within colleges and career training schools.
- Understand the benefits of timely submission of all required pre-externship paperwork and documentation.
- Identify the reasons why students should always present to their externship site with a résumé.
- Explain the typical process of submitting externship hours to the college for externship course attendance.
- Describe how your performance is linked to your final course grade.
- Identify miscellaneous requirements commonly imposed by colleges and schools.
- Describe the expected manner for handling communication issues regarding tardiness to or absence from the externship site.
- Identify the typical expectations of the externship site supervisor and staff/trainers concerning student externships.

Extern's Responsibility to Two Parties

In general, externs must fulfill the expectations of their academic institution and of their externship site supervisors and trainers. Meeting and exceeding expectations in both these areas are of equal importance. The best action you can take is to ask questions and be sure you have a thorough understanding of these expectations before the externship begins. Typically, an externship coordinator or other faculty member/instructor (perhaps with a differing title) from your school will be completely responsible for overseeing your externship phase. This person will also be the school's point of contact for your site supervisor.

Expectations of the School and Faculty

In most cases, pre-externship requirements concerning your student status with your school must be met first. These normally include a physical exam, a tuberculosis (TB) test, immunizations (especially for participation in clinical externships), student liability insurance, résumé and cover letter completion, and other professional and health requirements, such as a cardiopulmonary resuscitation (CPR) or basic life support (BLS) certification, and a practical skills competency check. Submitting your timesheet or record of hours as specified, maintaining contact with your faculty coordinator, and putting forth effort to learn are required throughout the externship.

Completing all externship requirements on time is extremely important. In addition to expected academic consequences, delays in beginning and completing the externship can have financial consequences (for those students receiving federal financial aid).

The following subsections pertain to your responsibilities to your academic institution and cover a wide variety of the requirements likely to be imposed by most colleges; however, each individual college/school has its own specific procedures and documentation requirements:

- Health documentation requirements
- Student liability coverage
- Career services department requirements
- Timesheets/record of externship hours submission
- The effort you expend
- Additional requirements

Health Documentation Requirements   For clinically oriented externship programs, almost every school stipulates a set of health/medical requirements and forms that students must complete prior to the externship start date. These vary by school but generally involve a comprehensive physical exam, along with certain immunizations/vaccinations and TB testing. Whatever the requirements are at your externship site, you must complete and submit this paperwork on time. The school/college will not allow students to participate in the externship without the required documentation. This involves advanced planning on your part, considering that you will probably have to wait to see a physician after you call to set an appointment to fulfill these requirements.

You should locate or obtain immunization records early in this process. This documentation is not always kept with current records and may require an extensive search, such as contacting a former family doctor or pediatrician for copies.

While completing these health requirements and before submitting them to your college, confirm that all information is legible and that all dates and signatures are visible. These documents (or copies of them) will be filed in your official student record.

Failure to supply all of this documentation will undoubtedly prevent you from beginning your externship, maintaining your status as a student-extern, and attending classes.

Student Liability Coverage   Another required item for your externship, which either will be your responsibility or will be provided by your school, is student professional liability insurance. Some schools subscribe to insurers that provide coverage for all students in specified programs. However, some schools require student-externs to purchase student professional liability insurance prior to their externship. If you do not know how this applies to you, you must ask your faculty adviser what is required. Although this is typically required and covered by the school, many externship site managers will not allow a student to begin the externship without proof of this insurance. Although this is both your school and site supervisors require this, it is only mentioned here to avoid repetitiveness.

Career Services Department Requirements   Many colleges, especially those with a career services/resources department, require students to complete a résumé, cover letter, and exit interview before graduating. These requirements may be due early when programs provide an externship at the conclusion of the program. Meeting your institution's due dates for graduation requirements ensures that you will gain at least three benefits: First, completing all paperwork ensures that you will not have any setbacks when it comes to receiving your official graduate status and diploma or degree; second, your career/employment services director/representative will have extra time to help you refine your résumé and to begin assisting you in your job search; and third, you will not have any documentation setbacks that would prevent you from beginning the externship on time. Beginning the externship late will likely delay your graduation date, and it may affect your externship course grade.

As noted, the résumé is an important document. It is to your benefit to take your completed, professional résumé to your externship site. For starters, it is the professional thing to do. This externship could be your first point of entry into the health care industry, so you should make your best first impression, even though technically you are still a student. Your résumé is useful for delineating previous jobs, responsibilities, and education, especially the allied health education you have been pursuing in recent months. Be sure to include any volunteer work, especially if it involves helping in a patient care setting of any sort. A detailed discussion of building an effective résumé is presented in Chapter Eleven of this text.

Submission of Timesheet or Record of Externship Hours   Timesheets or timecards for recording your externship hours can be handled in various ways. These may be given to you, or they may be distributed to your externship site supervisor directly by the externship faculty. If they are in your possession, be sure to keep them in a safe place. Once you officially begin the externship, ask your supervisor if there is a safe place in the office where you may store them. Slightly different procedures are imposed by different schools, but the main concept is that a clear and verifiable record of the hours you were present and participating at the site must be created. Typically, your hours will not be recognized as officially complete by your college until a signature or verbal verification of the supervisor, or both, is obtained by the school's externship coordinator. This is very important because the hours completed and submitted translate directly to your attendance record. It is to your benefit to keep a photocopy of these records, with signatures, as you would (and will) for an actual job. You may be instructed to fax your completed hours each week or so, or you may be required to physically take them to your school.

Both your externship coordinator and your site supervisor will expect you to handle the submission of your completed hours professionally; this includes being punctual, honest, and following appropriate procedures.

Unfortunately, some students are tempted to "fudge" a few hours here and there on their timesheet; however, anyone who has tried this has usually been caught and, when caught, has always been penalized. Because of the communication between the school's liaison or coordinator to the externship site and the staff at the site, false time credits are easily detectable. You should refrain from this type of dishonest behavior as it inevitably sets the stage for failure or some other negative consequence. It is also important to recognize that your externship site supervisor is *not* the person ultimately responsible for submitting your hours, unless this is arranged between your school faculty and the supervisor.

Remember: Abiding by the procedures related to timekeeping will help you to develop your abilities to be a responsible and accountable professional.

The Effort You Expend   You will, of course, be expected to perform your best and learn as you gain experience. Toward the end of your practical experience, your site supervisor and a faculty member from your school, or both, will evaluate you. Your college may request several periodic evaluations or just one on completion of your externship. Most colleges will determine your overall externship course grade based largely on how your supervisor rates you in these evaluations. Generally, a comprehensive evaluation form for a medical assisting externship includes specific competencies in the categories of clinical, practical, and administrative duties, as well as attributes of professionalism that you did or did not demonstrate while practicing. Similar organization applies to almost every allied health specialty. For example, administrative, professional, and practical skills are specified on evaluation forms for fields such as medical billing and coding, health information, pharmacy technology, dental hygiene, and so on. Knowing this, you probably will conclude that your externship should be taken seriously and demands the professionalism of an actual job. If possible, request from your program faculty a sample copy of the evaluation form by which your performance will be rated. Use this form for reference before and throughout your externship. You can use the evaluation as a pre-externship preparation tool to identify technical skills or competencies for which you feel you need extra practice or review before going to practice in the field. Chapter 9 contains more information concerning how you will be evaluated, along with a few sample evaluation forms.

Additional Requirements   Prior to the practicum, your school may have some additional requirements. For example, the individual departments within your school may have to sign certain paperwork to demonstrate that you have met their respective requirements for graduation. It is likely that you will have to be trained in CPR, first aid, and/or BLS before the externship, with your valid certification card serving as proof of completion. Once you have fulfilled this requirement and received a certification card, be sure to submit a copy for your student file and to include the certification and effective date on your résumé.

You may also be required to provide written or signed verification from your clinical instructor(s)/faculty to indicate that you have mastered all skill areas relevant to your program. This is particularly important for medical assistants and other clinically trained students attempting to complete an accredited program. Many schools have an established practical skills test that students must pass to prove competency prior to the externship. Even if this is not a stipulated requirement at your school or college, you should still seek verification by your instructors, for your own benefit, that you are completely competent in all skills. In addition, it may be required that student-externs undergo a drug test, a background check, or both prior to the externship. This requirement can be imposed by either your school or the externship site.

Communication on a regular basis with your supervising faculty or externship coordinator is vital. If you have any days during which you are ill or have a valid excuse for arriving late to the site, you must call your site and you must speak to or at least leave a message for your school's coordinator concerning the situation. It is imperative that both your coordinator and site manager are informed of this situation at the same time. Contact the site supervisor as soon as possible, just as you would for an actual job. If the externship site was your employer and you failed to report with a timely phone call that you would not be showing up for work, you might not have that job by day's end. Externs have been dismissed from their externship sites for not arriving as scheduled and failing to make contact with a phone call. On the first day of your externship, ask your site supervisor what additional steps are required beyond these basic notification procedures in the case that you will be late or unable to attend. Be sure to keep the appropriate telephone number readily available in case you need it.

You are expected to take responsibility and communicate appropriately in all such cases. The communication skills you exhibit are a significant indicator of your overall level of professionalism.

In summary, prior to your externship date you should verify with your externship coordinator that everything you must do is officially completed prior to your externship start date. If you find yourself lagging in doing this, realize that finalizing these requirements on time will save you the time and stress it takes to get them done at the last minute.

Expectations of the Externship Site Staff and Trainers

The following points, which pertain to general expectations of the professionals working on site with student-externs during the externship, are discussed throughout the following subsections.

• Punctuality and effective communication
• Proactive learning
• Adaptability in the workplace
• Willingness to cross-train
• Recognition of protective measures for health care workers

Punctuality and Effective Communication   When physician offices or other medical facilities agree to provide a training atmosphere for new allied health workers, they agree to it with several expectations of you, the student. Your trainers will expect you to arrive as scheduled (on time) and work your full shift productively with the intent to work and learn. Your supervisor or trainer expects you to be as professional as the rest of the staff. One expectation is that, for the short term of your externship, there should be no absences or tardiness issues. Not arriving as scheduled and being late convey lack of professionalism and lack of a work ethic. If there must be an absence, normal professional protocol, as described previously in this chapter, should be followed. Make telephone contact ahead of time; do not waltz through the door late, even if it is only five minutes late, without a phone call, and then expect no consequences. Even if your site seems to be a friendly and comfortable environment, where being late may not seem detrimental to daily operations, somebody will always take notice, especially if these events are habitual throughout your externship.

 HIGHLIGHT: Tips from Professionals

"Treat your externship like a real job. This is the career you have chosen; therefore, you should treat it in that manner. . . . Set a regular schedule, show up on the days to which you have committed, and show up on time. If you cannot attend, call the office and leave a message. Come prepared, ready to work and learn. Take your externship seriously and be professional."

Stephanie Riley
Front Office Coordinator, Pediatrics Office

Proactive Learning Two specific areas regarding the expectation that you must "work your full shift productively with intent to learn" merit further explanation. First, the word *full* describing *shift* means that leaving earlier than scheduled is unacceptable, with the exception of a true emergency. As always, somebody will observe your actions. The other key term is *productively.* While at the externship site, you are expected, at the very least, to do the following: be proactive in your learning and take initiative. To learn proactively, you must participate by taking notes, keeping a journal, asking questions, volunteering, and so on, even during a slow time of day. Those training you will see this as professional on your part; it shows them you are motivated, interested in your field of study, and trainable. Your diligence to learn proactively may be a heavily weighted factor in a supervisor's decision to hire you. Once you are familiar with the workings of the facility to which you are assigned, you should be exhibiting initiative to keep up the pace. At no time of day should you be doing nothing. Never sit around and wait to be told what to do, and never use slow times to catch up on your nonexternship business, like reading magazines, listening to personal voice mail and returning phone calls, e-mailing, and the like. At such times, ask what you can do to help in another area of the office, even if it's cleaning up or reorganizing the office desk or patient waiting area. Your initiative will impress managers and potential employers because it shows that you work with a caring and positive attitude.

Adaptability in the Workplace Another professional skill that site staff will expect you to demonstrate is *adaptability.* How easily can you adapt to change? If a new manager takes over your externship site while you are on the externship, and your duties are suddenly more varied than before, can you handle it? Furthermore, can you handle it *professionally?* What if new software for the office is implemented while you are on your externship, once you just finished learning the old system? What if another employee is on leave for a week due to illness or surgery, and the manager asks you to come in an hour earlier each day of that week to help carry the workload? Most people would agree that these tasks are doable. However, changes may occur at an unexpected or inopportune time. This can be irritating if it inconveniences you. Nonetheless, if you must face the challenge of change, the professional way to handle it is to willingly cooperate with the rest of

HIGHLIGHT: Tips from Professionals

"Treat your externship like you would study for a test. Take good notes during your shifts and when you go home, review, review, review."

Natasha Smith
Medical Assistant, Electrophysiology (EP) Department, Multi-Facility Cardiology Practice

the team. It is even more important to do so without complaining, while exhibiting a positive attitude and professionalism. Change in the workplace is inevitable, so exercising your flexibility in this area during the externship, if necessary, will benefit you.

Willingness to Cross-Train   Even if you have been educated in only one concentration or discipline, your site manager will likely have a system of cross-training prepared for you. Medical assistants especially should expect to take part in cross-training during the externship. Whatever the case, you must be prepared to accept the breadth of the training you are given. For example, you may be preparing for an externship in medical assisting and your favorite tasks are to perform phlebotomies and administer injections; however, the site manager is planning that you will complete a schedule of mornings working one-on-one with patients in the back office and performing certain clinical tasks, then spending afternoons assisting and learning such front office tasks as scheduling, filing insurance claims, ordering labs and prescriptions. Although students typically prefer certain tasks to others, your training program must be comprehensive, and it is to your benefit to gladly receive the training offered in all areas. For medical assistants engaging in externship under American Association of Medical Assistants (AAMA) regulations, specific division of front and back office experience is a requirement. For future employment purposes, you will be able to document this cross-training experience, if applicable, on your post-externship résumé. The training staff also expects you to be willing to learn in this way.

Another benefit of cross-training during your externship is that you will understand how your specific tasks and responsibilities contribute to the overall functioning of the externship site. Gaining this perspective will help you professionally since your understanding will lead to increased effectiveness in your specialty.

Recognition of Protective Measures for Health Care Workers   For clinically trained externs, the site supervisor will likely assume that you are well aware of the Bloodborne Pathogens Standard of the Occupational Safety and Health Administration (OSHA) and the Universal Precautions of the Centers for Disease Control (CDC). If you feel you do not know or have forgotten any of the specifics related to these standards, you must master them prior to your externship. Your externship site will have a way for you to access this information. However, do not arrive at your site without a general knowledge of what the regulations cover and why they exist. In addition, be sure you remember the guidelines covering the use of personal protective equipment (PPE).

Obviously, these regulations and guidelines are more applicable in some facilities than they are in others; for instance, in an outpatient surgical center or dental specialty facility, these would be referenced much more often than they would in a primary care office, a claims processing office, or a retail pharmacy. Also, some professionals will not observe these guidelines if their particular work within the facility does not call for adherence to them; for instance, the human resources (HR) office employees of a large medical group or hospital, or the business manager of an outpatient surgical center, would not be in appropriate positions to follow the Bloodborne Pathogen Standard, the Universal Precautions, or the use of PPE. By the time you begin your externship, you should know the extent to which these guidelines apply to your specific function within allied health.

Going Above and Beyond

You can go above and beyond all expectations by preparing yourself for your career after the externship. Joining a professional organization and preparing yourself for certification can help demonstrate your commitment to the allied health field.

Join a Professional Organization as a Student Member

While completing your coursework, apply for student membership in a professional organization for your chosen field. You can document this membership on your résumé, and this will communicate to the health care community that you are dedicated to becoming a fully qualified professional. It shows your externship supervisor and potential employers that you have joined your peers in a professional association and are being exposed through that organization to the most recent standards, advancements, and ethical requirements in the field.

Prepare Early for Registration and Certification in Your Profession

Become certified or registered in your profession prior to beginning your externship. Generally, applications to sit for these various credentialing exams are due well in advance of the actual test date. Planning ahead is necessary if you wish to become professionally credentialed within a reasonable period after graduation. Your allied health department faculty should be able to direct you to the appropriate point of contact for obtaining application materials, or your school may deal directly with some of these organizations to provide on-site testing. Once you have obtained the registration materials, carefully consider the test date for which you will be eligible, and take note of the application due date and any additional documentation requirements for completion of your application. For example, some of the organizations require references or letters of recommendation, along with your basic application form. Make note of the registration fee for the exam, as payment must be submitted with your application for it to be processed. (See Appendix: Selected Allied-Health Certification and Credentialing Resources at the end of this text for a listing of allied health professional organizations, the certification/registration each awards, and Web site information.)

CONCLUSION

Aligning yourself with the expectations discussed in this chapter will ensure success both in relationship to your dealings with your faculty coordinator and your externship site supervisor(s). Maintain a steady focus in these areas. It is possible to be dismissed from the externship position by the supervising staff member or manager due to professional inadequacies; it has happened to students before, but fortunately it is easily preventable. Many more professional attributes that externship site managers, staff trainers, and physicians expect are described throughout the remainder of this text. Continue to use this guide to evaluate yourself prior to the externship so that you are well prepared for a positive and productive experience.

Self-Prep Questions

1. Do you have a particular interest regarding the medical specialty or type of facility in which you would like to work? Write down your interests and communicate them to your externship coordinator in advance of your externship. Also communicate your interests to your school's career services staff.

   I would like to work in a larger facility, maybe oncology, or end of life care, but I am very interested in working in a phlebotomy clinic, depending on how that class goes.

2. Acquire or make a list of your school's health (and any other) requirements that must be complete before the externship. How far in advance does documentation need to be submitted?

   Background checks
   TB panel update

_____

_____

_____

_____

_____

_____

3. Write down the contact information for your externship coordinator, school/college, and medical/health instructors. Include fax number(s).

_____

_____

_____

_____

_____

_____

_____

_____

4. How will your attendance and hours be monitored by your institution? What specific responsibilities are yours concerning submission of your hours?

_____

_____

_____

_____

_____

_____

_____

_____

5. Make a list of any skills you need to practice more. Be sure to communicate these needs to your faculty/instructors at an appropriate time prior to the externship.

accurately obtaining BP

6. Recall a situation in class, at a job, or elsewhere in which you had to quickly adapt to a new way of doing things. If you cannot recall one of your own personal experiences, create a medical office scenario that includes a significant change and explain how you, the extern, should adapt.

QVC - new RF guns

Role-Play Scenario

Two or more individuals are needed for this scenario. Suppose the externship coordinator (one of the individuals) is presenting the pre-externship requirements of your school to a group of externs beginning externship in the near future. The externship coordinator should review all school requirements for this group with basic instructions. The group/audience (the other one or more individuals) must each ask at least two questions of the acting externship coordinator about different topics or requirements she or he presents. Members of the group or audience should ask questions that test the knowledge of the externship coordinator, and the coordinator should ask questions and request solutions of group members regarding, for example, how to follow basic procedures, resolve problematic situations, or compile pre-externship documents and other requirements. This exercise is intended to help participating individuals to gain a better understanding of their school's specific externship requirements.

1. What are the main topics the externship coordinator would need to cover for the presentation, based on your school/college's externship requirements?

_____

_____

_____

_____

_____

_____

_____

_____

_____

_____

2. What are some details concerning some of the points made that the group can ask questions about?

_____

_____

_____

_____

_____

_____

_____

_____

_____

3. How can the externship coordinator make sure that the group has a thorough understanding of the requirements?

_____

_____

_____

_____

_____

_____

_____

_____

_____

Readiness Checklist

_____ I know what documentation is required of my institution's program prior to beginning the externship.

_____ I know the timeframe and due dates I must meet to accomplish timely submission of these requirements.

_____ I am aware of the issue with student liability insurance, and I know whether I am responsible for this or whether my school provides appropriate coverage.

_____ I understand the method of hours (attendance) submission to which I am expected to abide, and I understand the consequences of not following the appropriate procedures.

_____ I understand my program's method of evaluating my performance throughout the externship.

_____ I have received verification by my classroom and lab instructors that I am competent in my technical skills and knowledge.

___✓___ I understand the importance of appropriate communication with my faculty or externship coordinator and with my externship site staff trainers.

___✓___ I understand the minimum expectations of the externship site managers and trainers who agree to train me at their facility.

___✓___ I understand that my absences and/or tardiness should be nonexistent unless an emergency is pending. If I must be absent or late, I understand the typical professional protocol for communicating this to my externship site supervisor.

✓ I understand that I am expected to work my full shift and to do so productively.

✓ I have identified what it means to adapt professionally to change when necessary.

✓ I understand that rather than repeating my favorite skills during my externship, I may be assigned to learn the tasks of other areas in the office or facility. It is evident to me why this cross-training may be expected and also why it works to my advantage.

✓ I have read and understand the content of the OSHA Bloodborne Pathogens Standard and the CDC's Universal Precautions.

✓ I understand the benefits of joining a professional organization as a student member.

chapter three

Externship Interviews

Introduction

Many externship site managers request to meet with or interview potential student-externs prior to officially accepting the externship in their facilities. In the eyes of managers, this often is necessary because these professionals, while accommodating an extern, still have to manage operations and account for the productivity of their facilities or departments while using time and resources to help students meet externship objectives. Most would like to be certain in advance that the student is able to work professionally and is competent in the skills necessary to practice in the facility.

Prior to officially accepting an externship, site managers and supervisors learn what they need to know about students by gathering relevant information and conducting interviews, during which they form first impressions. This chapter explores why such interviews may be required, and it describes numerous ways that the student can prepare for and do well in the interview. The chapter concludes with Self-Prep Questions, a Role-Play Scenario, and a Readiness Checklist.

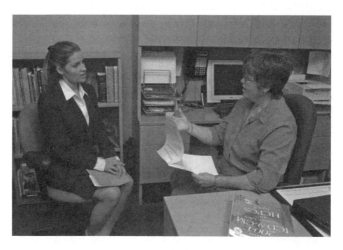

In attending an interview for the externship, it is important to appear professional, as well as to demonstrate confidence, interest, and a positive attitude.

Chapter Objectives

- Identify three reasons why many facility supervisors request an interview or preliminary meeting with the extern candidate prior to accepting the externship.
- Identify the possible ways a student can research (or at least become familiar with) a medical practice or health care company prior to meeting or interviewing with the manager.
- List at least seven intelligent interview questions a student-extern can ask the interviewer when prompted.
- Specify the importance of arriving at the externship site with a professional résumé in hand.
- List at least nine rules of thumb concerning professional appearance for the interview and the externship.
- Name three practices to adhere to during the interview or preliminary meeting.
- Describe the proper method of establishing the externship schedule with the site manager if special scheduling is necessary.

Requests for an Externship Interview

You may or may not be asked to participate in an interview for your externship. The requirement depends on the preference of the site manager who will be allowing you to practice your skills in his or her office. Some feel comfortable with any capable student walking into the office with no contact prior to the day he or she is supposed to begin the externship. On the other hand, many others are a bit more particular about this and feel more comfortable meeting the student on site for an interview before officially accepting him or her for the externship. Therefore, you should be prepared for this type of professional meeting. It is also possible that you may obtain a job directly through your externship, and an externship interview may be the first step in that direction.

Reasons for a Preliminary Interview

For various specific reasons, a site manager may request an interview or some other type of introductory meeting prior to your starting the externship. First, an interview with the student helps the manager to assess at least three major characteristics: how well you communicate and present yourself; what professional qualities you exhibit; and how well you are likely to perform the clinical, administrative, and other practical duties specific to your specialty. These particular aspects are very important to the manager because you will be a representative of his or her organization if you are accepted for the externship.

The managing staff also may request to meet with you first to provide you with a tour of the facility, to show you the various areas in which you will be working as an extern. Some offices already have a system established in all areas of their offices with which they train all externs, and they may use this meeting time as an opportunity to explain their particular system of training to you.

This time also may be used to introduce you to other office staff who may take part in training you. As you know by now, your first in-person encounter gives the all-important first impression of you to the interviewer. Therefore, it is crucial that you consider in advance how you will present yourself with a positive attitude, confidence, and professionalism. As always, it is up to you to present your best in any meeting or interview.

Proactive Measures for Externship Interviews

The bulk of the material presented in this chapter informs you about the ways in which you can prepare yourself to make a favorable first impression in an externship interview. The remaining sections cover the following considerations:

- Researching the site
- Submitting your résumé
- Completing application and information forms
- Presenting yourself as a professional
- Discussing your availability and setting a schedule

Researching the Site

If the medical office or facility maintains an informative Web site about the practice or company, visit the site and commit to memory such details as the daily hours of operation, additional office locations, the number of doctors who practice on site, which medical specialties are practiced in the office, and so on. This will prepare you to ask intelligent questions of the interviewer about the staff and the organization. It also will help you demonstrate your general interest in the patient care industry. Perhaps of greatest significance to the interviewing manager or staff, it will illustrate a certain level of professionalism on your part that you intentionally researched the organization before interviewing.

Typically, in interviews of any kind, you will be asked what questions, if any, you have for the interviewer. You must avoid answering "None" when this is asked. Always be prepared to ask at least one or two intelligent questions. Save any questions that focus on you for the end of your interview. The following questions will suffice in a medical setting:

- How long have the physicians at this office been practicing?
- Do the physicians practice in this office only, or do they also see patients in a hospital or at another site?
- What procedures are performed routinely in this office?

- How many patients are seen on a daily basis by each practitioner?
- In addition to the physicians, what other patient care professionals work in the office (e.g., physician assistants, nurse practitioners, registered nurses, medical assistants, X-ray technicians)?
- What specific credentials do you seek when you hire for a medical assisting (or other allied health, etc.) career position?
- Should you decide to accept me as an extern, what are the main areas of your facility in which I will be assisting while I am completing my externship hours?

Submitting Your Résumé

The first day you set foot in a possible or established externship site, you should have a résumé in hand to provide to the office manager. Prior to that, take advantage of the résumé writing and career development resources available at your school. Your résumé is especially important because it often will determine the first impression of you a potential employer will develop. So, seek all the advice available to you regarding the building of a professional résumé. You will demonstrate forethought and professionalism when you have your résumé available for the externship site manager when you first meet. For specific details on building an effective résumé, see Chapter Eleven.

Completing Application and Information Forms

The manager you meet for an interview may ask you to complete an employment application. Do not assume that this means you will be hired when you complete your externship. Oftentimes, managers who request this of you basically prefer to see all your information in the format to which they are accustomed, knowing that it will give them the information they need. At some future time it may serve as an actual employment application, but you cannot count on this. All you can know is that the manager may or may not intend to hire you in the future and that you are expected to complete the application professionally. If this request is made of you, complete the form(s) thoroughly, accurately, and legibly.

Presenting Yourself as a Professional

Your goal in any interview, whether for externship or employment, is to make a positive and lasting first impression. Concerning appearances, in the medical setting it is essential to maintain personal cleanliness and professional grooming. When interviewing for an externship as a student, you may be able to wear the uniform or scrubs and student ID that are required by your academic program, or you may be required to dress in more generic interview attire. Always check with your faculty or externship coordinator regarding the dress standards your training institution requires for an externship interview. The following tips apply to your externship interview:

- Your scrubs (and lab coat, if required) should be clean and wrinkle free.
- Perfume should be avoided, as some patients or staff members may have allergies or sensitivities that are irritated by fragrances.
- Makeup should be kept to a minimum. Dangling, distracting, noisy jewelry should not be worn; only very small earrings, wedding rings, and wristwatches are appropriate.
- If your hair is longer than shoulder length, it should be tied back neatly and securely.
- Nails should be neat, clean, and short. Artificial nails are generally not acceptable due to their tendency to harbor bacteria.
- Shoes should be clean, without holes, tears, or excessive scuffing.
- As a rule of thumb, body piercing in odd places (nose, chin, tongue, eyebrow, etc.) and tattoos should not be visible.

These pointers may seem elementary, but you must abide by them in any professional medical facility.

You should also use your manners, express a desire to learn, and remember the name of the person with whom you have interviewed. Communicating in a courteous manner contributes to your overall professional demeanor. Any hint of an unappreciative attitude gives a first impression that is difficult to erase. Showing the medical staff member(s) that you are excited about the opportunity to learn in their office will gain for you their professional respect and willingness to help you learn as much as possible. Of course, it never fails that some students forget the name of their interviewer(s). The best and most professional way to avoid this pitfall is to obtain and study a business card while you are on site for an externship interview or for your first day working as a student-extern.

 HIGHLIGHT: Tips from Professionals

"About first impressions. . . . Appropriate dress is important. Also, tattoos must be covered and body piercings and jewelry taken out. In one instance, I could not accept a student for a position simply because of a tattoo on her wrist."

Denise Wenger
Office Manager, OB/GYN Group Practice

Timely arrival for your scheduled interview is also part of the first impression you give the site supervisor or interviewer. It is best to arrive approximately ten minutes prior to the interview. Also, if you do not know exactly where the site is located, map it out a few days before your appointment so that you will not arrive late. Also, consider traffic patterns in your locality in determining how much time you will need to arrive on time. Demonstrating punctuality as part of your overall first impression is a necessity.

Discussing Your Availability and Setting a Schedule

Some students need to balance the externship with another job or unavoidable responsibility. While such occurrences are inevitable, it is important to make yourself as available and as flexible as possible for scheduling unless your school or college specifies that a full-time or other preestablished schedule must be met. It is important to let the site supervisor or interviewer know ahead of time if you will need a unique set of hours for your externship; politely ask if he or she would be willing to accommodate you in this circumstance. You must discuss this ahead of time so that the site staff is not expecting you to conform to a schedule that you cannot possibly meet.

Many of the managers who agree to have students in the office understand the expense of being a student and that it may be necessary for the student to keep an additional job to maintain income. When attempting to schedule the maximum number of hours you think you can handle, be realistic in considering your other priorities so you do not overestimate your availability and then have to ask for a reduced schedule. Work out a schedule with the site supervisor in advance of the first day of the externship. Once you have agreed to it, get it approved by your externship coordinator.

HIGHLIGHT: Tips from Professionals

- During an externship interview, be sure to be on time, dress to impress, leave kids with a baby-sitter, be mindful of perfume and jewelry, and turn off the cell phone or leave it in the car.
- Be on time.
- Dress to impress.
- Leave kids with a babysitter.
- Be mindful of perfume and jewelry.
- Turn off the cell phone or leave it in the car.

Natasha Smith,
Medical Assistant, Electrophysiology (EP) Department,
Multi-Facility Cardiology Practice

Keep in mind that you typically have to complete your hours within a predetermined timeframe, so careful planning is necessary. Your externship syllabus and other paperwork may specify a certain number of hours weekly; if this is the case, plan according to these requirements, too. Of course, occasional times of hardship or illness leave a student no choice but to be absent from the externship for a short period of time. Thus it is important to prepare a backup plan for quickly making up any hours missed. Ask the site supervisor if, in the event of such a situation, you will be able to have an additional week on site to make up time. While dealing with everyday life, it remains very important to treat the externship with as much priority and care as your other responsibilities, keeping in mind that it is another opportunity to make a favorable impression.

Going Above and Beyond

Prior to attending an externship interview, go a step further to improve the interviewer's overall impression of you. Discuss with your instructors which certification exams you will be eligible to sit for on completion of your program. Know the name of the agency that awards the certification, as well as the exact name and official abbreviation of the certification itself (e.g., CMA, RMA, NCMA, NCMOA, RHIT, CPC, RPT, NCET, etc.). Determine when you will be able to take a certification exam (see Chapter 2). When the time comes for you to discuss your professional goals with your interviewer, by prepared to describe your plans. The interviewer will then recognize your commitment to your specialty and your professional planning. (See the Appendix for the titles, abbreviations, and Web site addresses of credentialing agencies.)

CONCLUSION

Your overall goal for an externship interview or another type of pre-externship meeting with the site manager is to make an excellent first impression so that the site staff will willingly accommodate you in their office. A positive first impression will get you off to a good start. A catchy, clear, and impressively assembled résumé will help with the first impression your interviewer forms. Be prepared with your résumé, be somewhat familiar with the facility and how it operates, and be ready to share your own professional goals confidently.

Self-Prep Questions

1. In addition to the questions cited in this chapter, what are some other intelligent questions you might ask the interviewer if you have an externship interview?

_____

_____

_____

_____

_____

_____

_____

_____

2. Write down the resources available to you that will assist you in creating a professional résumé and in performing successfully in an interview.

_____

_____

_____

_____

_____

_____
_____
_____
_____

3. Critique yourself based on past interviews or any professional encounters, or ask a peer to take you through a mock interview. Recognize and list which aspects of interviewing are your strengths and which are your weaknesses. Think of ways to improve these weaknesses.

_____
_____
_____
_____
_____
_____
_____
_____
_____

Role-Play Scenario

Two individuals are needed for this scenario. Perform a five- to ten-minute role-play in which the interviewer asks an extern candidate relevant questions about his or her experience, training, goals for the externship, professional goals, and so on. The student-extern being interviewed should demonstrate a working understanding of how to create a good first impression through this interview.

1. Make a list of common interview questions (regardless of specialty), as well as a list of questions tailored to the externship specialty that an interviewer can pose. Approximately five questions for each of these two areas will suffice.

_____
_____
_____

_____

_____

_____

_____

_____

_____

_____

_____

_____

_____

_____

2. List the key areas the student-extern candidate must consider and present during this interview process to make a positive first impression.

_____

_____

_____

_____

_____

_____

_____

_____

_____

_____

Readiness Checklist

_____ I am prepared for an externship interview if I am asked to attend one.

_____ I understand why an externship site manager probably will request an interview or preliminary meeting.

_____ I understand the benefits of researching a medical practice or company prior to the interview.

_____ I have committed to memory at least three intelligent questions to ask an interviewer.

_____ I have or will have my résumé prepared and updated in time for an externship interview.

_____ I understand the basic physical appearance guidelines for the interview and the entire externship.

_____ I understand that during the interview I am expected to be well mannered and to demonstrate interest in learning more about my field.

_____ I will make it a point to remember the name of the person with whom I interview and to request a business card.

_____ I will discuss with the site manager, in advance of the externship, any special scheduling arrangements I will need once I am accepted for the externship. I understand that this also must be communicated to and approved by the externship coordinator.

chapter four

Attitudes and Perceptions

Introduction

Perhaps the phrase "Attitude is everything" is familiar to you. People say it because attitudes profoundly influence one's success in most areas of life, especially in the professional world. Perceptions are precursors of the specific attitudes people possess. This chapter explains the connection between perceptions and attitudes and presents the most applicable recommendations and warnings as far as both are concerned. Attitudes that can ruin the externship experience are presented with descriptions of how they can become detrimental. Positive and professionally effective attitudes can shape a productive and rewarding externship, and these are identified with descriptions of how they can lead to success during the externship, as well as during your career. The chapter concludes with Self-Prep Questions, a Role-Play Scenario, and a Readiness Checklist.

(a)

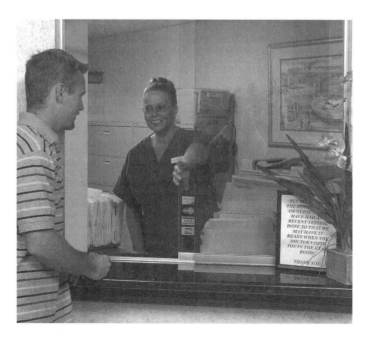

(b)

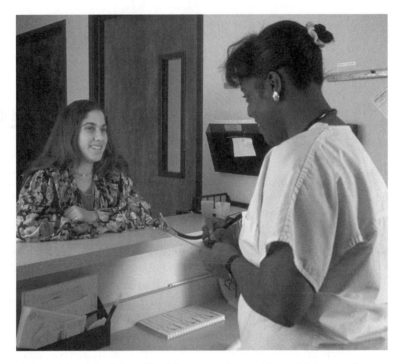

Figure 4-1 (a) and (b)   Health care workers with positive attitudes and smiling faces contribute to patient satisfaction and cooperation.

Chapter Objectives

- List five general characteristics that contribute to an overall positive attitude.
- List five general characteristics that reflect an overall negative attitude.
- List at least five detrimental perceptions and attitudes a student might possess.
- Explain how each of the five detrimental attitudes can affect overall professional effectiveness.
- List at least four positive attitudes a student should demonstrate during the externship.
- Explain how those four positive attitudes affect overall professional effectiveness.

Attitude and the Allied Health Externship

Attitude is one of the most significant factors of professional success. The attitude you portray can communicate much about you, both positive and negative. This self-portrayal (defined only by you) can lead you to a fantastic start at your

HIGHLIGHT: Tips from Professionals

"Personality is very important, especially when dealing with patients (customers). . . . You must have a pleasant attitude and be outgoing."

Paula Kennell,
Office Manager, Family Medicine Practice

externship site, or it can be the beginning of a downward spiral that may get you dismissed. A positive attitude in your externship environment is characterized by optimism, friendliness, confidence, willingness to learn and gain experience in all areas of the facility, and appreciation for the training and experience provided to you. Excessive pessimism, complaining, grumpiness, self-pity, indifference, and arrogance reflect an all-around negative attitude. Contrary to the belief of some pessimists, attitudes can be changed for the better. Let's see how.

Recognizing the Human Nature of Perceptions and Attitudes

Where does an attitude come from? An experience, an expectation, someone else's influence, the media, another source? Underlying any attitude is at least one perception, which is simply your viewpoint or interpretation of an object, idea, person or circumstance. For example, what is your attitude toward your education? How is this attitude shaped? You might agree that it is shaped mostly by how you feel about your instructors, your peers, the structure and content of the course material, and the learning environment. External factors outside your educational experience, such as how you view life and other people in general, can also play a role in your attitude toward your education.

The way you see or construe your life experiences fosters the attitudes you currently hold in regard to your school or college. For example, if you feel uncomfortable with your instructors and your learning style does not mesh with their teaching methods, then you likely have an attitude of doubt and disdain. On the other hand, if your experience has been positive, with a well-equipped learning environment and instructors with whom you can relate and whose instruction you can grasp, then your attitude is likely positive, which results in personal benefit to you: You are confident, motivated, and feel you are progressing steadily and successfully in accomplishing your goals. Thus, it is necessary for you to be aware of how your perceptions influence your overall attitude.

The following are some of the many synonyms that show the close relation of the terms *perception* and *attitude*. Occasionally the two are actually used as synonyms for each other; however, this analysis differentiates the two in order to observe the more outward aspect of the term *attitude* relative to the more internal aspect of *perception:*

Perception   conception, image, impression, viewpoint, insight
Attitude   character, demeanor, inclination, temperament, mental state

Attitudes are interesting because people can interpret them based on a number of features. Attitudes can be reflected by facial expressions, tone of voice, choice of words, physical mannerisms, and general behavior. Considering your upcoming entry into the health care setting, it is important that you realize that people can typically perceive attitudes in one form or another. Considering that these attitudes are determined by underlying perceptions, the starting point to change any bad attitudes for the better is through a change in perception. Some changes in this area can be challenging; others may be fairly simple. No scientific formula can be followed to change people's perceptions because each person is unique in this dimension of the mind. The bottom line is that in order to change an existing "bad" perception, one must first recognize the need for the change and possess motivation to change it. This works most of the time when the person realizes it is to his or her own benefit to adopt more positive interpretations of his or her life situations, while letting go of the negative perceptions that cripple his or her chances of success. As a student-extern, it is to your benefit personally and professionally to examine your attitudes and trace those needing improvement to the perceptions that shape them.

This chapter first discusses what specific perceptions and attitudes are detrimental, followed by a discussion of those you can acquire that will lead you to success at your site. As you read, keep in mind that those attitudes you portray can positively or negatively influence your success in working with medical professionals and patients.

Changing Detrimental Attitudes and Perceptions

To get the most out of your externship, it is important to have the right attitude. Thus, certain perceptions will be detrimental to you and your experience, so you should avoid them. The following are examples of such perceptions.

Detrimental Perception #1: "I provide free labor."

You must not believe during the externship that you provide free labor for someone's business. Convincing yourself of this false notion will damage your overall attitude. For one thing, "unpaid" externships are mandated by some accrediting and credentialing agencies, such as the AAMA. Also, during your externship, you are not doing the site staff a favor; rather, the site staff are doing you a favor. During this phase, you are not considered to be an independent, qualified professional since you do not yet possess an adequate level of experience. You have not even graduated officially from your program, and chances are that you have not yet had the opportunity to sit for a credentialing exam.

The externship is an integral part of your training, and you are the one with the most to gain from it. And due to the initial training that must be provided, an externship often reduces the staff's productivity. You should view your externship as the site staff's sacrifice for your benefit, and you should express an attitude of gratitude. Your trainers and supervisors will quickly sense whether your attitude is positive or negative.

The following constitutes the components of this detrimental perception:

- *The detrimental perception:* "I am free labor. This manager only wants to use me for free work. Why should I work for free?"
- *Signs of the detrimental attitude:* Outward signs of dismay, such as a disgruntled demeanor and lack of motivation.
- *The realization:* "This supervisor or staff member is taking time out to help me learn and be successful. It is a good and charitable work for managers and employees to agree to help new budding allied health professionals gain appropriate experience."
- *The good perception:* "I see the value in what I am being offered through the externship and will appreciate it and take with me new experiences necessary for my professional growth."
- *Signs of a good attitude:* Willingness to learn, satisfaction in the externship experience, resulting in a happy vibe, thankfulness to those helping you, and good customer service.

Detrimental Perception #2: "I performed well in school, so I am an expert."

The belief that you have already mastered and become an expert in your respective allied health specialty just because you performed well in school is another perception that will not earn you one iota of respect. You have many practical lessons (both technical and professional) to learn during the externship. This is not to be confused with possessing confidence in your work; display confidence by all means, but not a know-it-all or haughty attitude. Yes, you deserve much credit for your classroom attendance and hard-earned grades, but this is far from the completion of your education.

You should pursue the externship for what it truly is: another new course in your curriculum. Look carefully at your school's course description for the externship. Also read the syllabus for the course objectives and description of what is expected of you, as you would for any course. Only after you successfully complete the externship should you pat yourself on the back for completing the full spectrum of your training.

Furthermore, you may choose to obtain an even higher qualification that will prove your expertise: that is, one or more of several credentialing and certification exams. Even beyond this, nothing on paper (certificates, diplomas, degrees, or professional memberships) compares to the expertise of an experienced professional. Once you achieve that level, which takes much time and hard work, then you will have good reason to consider yourself a fully qualified professional or expert in your field. When you eventually become a credentialed and experienced professional, be sure that your success does not prompt you to form an attitude of arrogance because it will surely diminish your professional reputation.

The following constitutes the components of this detrimental perception:

- *The detrimental perception:* "I already know everything I need to know. There is not much the externship experience can offer me."

- *Signs of the detrimental attitude:* The haughty, know-it-all attitude, which others see as arrogance; cannot take constructive criticism; difficult to function as a team player; irritation when others try to help you.

- *The realization:* "The externship is a new experience, where my skills will be tested and refined in a real-world setting with genuine professionals. It will be completely different from the classroom experience and a beneficial challenge."

- *The good perception:* "I will be around real professionals I can admire. They will help me to cultivate the professionalism expected in this field and to further refine my skills. This is all to my benefit."

- *Signs of a good attitude:* Confidence in existing skills, readiness to ask for advice to improve your skills, and finding value in what your peers and supervisor(s) contribute to your learning.

Detrimental Perception #3: "Externship? Whatever. . . ."

A laissez-faire attitude is unacceptable. If you demonstrate a blasé mind-set, those supervising you will know that you are not interested in what you are doing and that you will not be a valuable asset to their team, or to any other medical team or office to which they might otherwise refer you for future employment. If you are the type of student who is overly relaxed or indifferent, with no sense of urgency when it comes to getting tasks done in a timely manner, and getting them done right, then you should ponder this aspect of yourself and devise a plan for improvement. Medical offices and other facilities are typically in hustle mode each and every day as they tend to patients and customers. An extra body has no business lingering unproductively on site when a busy schedule must be met. Students can be and have been dismissed from sites for showing this nonchalant and disinterested attitude. (Remember that dismissal from a site will impact your grade.)

Indifference is also an attitude that can be easily detected in any type of interview or first meeting, so consider this ahead of time. It may be comfortable for you to take your time doing things, with no sense of urgency, and there may be nothing wrong with this as a personality trait and during your leisure time. However, in patient care and customer-focused facilities, this cannot be the attitude you present, whether as a student-extern or an employee. Productivity is expected no matter what area of allied health you are pursuing.

The following constitutes the components of this detrimental perception:

- *The detrimental perception:* "This is boring. Oh well, whatever, there's no hurry. I'll just wait until somebody gives me instructions. It does not really matter what I do anyway, as long as I am at the site."
- *Signs of the detrimental attitude:* Disinterest in your career field, lack of initiative or drive to work, appearing lazy or bored or both.
- *The realization:* "There is no tolerance for laziness or lack of productivity in patient care. Nobody will consider employing a person demonstrating these characteristics, not to mention consideration for career promotion."
- *The good perception:* "There is a standard of care and professionalism that must be maintained, and I will rise to the challenge of the rapid pace and diligence involved in all areas of health care."
- *Signs of a good attitude:* Readiness to work, efficient and effective work habits, asking questions and seeking advice, taking the initiative in all possible situations, offering help to others.

Detrimental Perception #4: "My personal problems are more than I can manage today."

Arriving to work with an obviously grumpy or unhappy attitude due to personal problems will be noticed, and you will be perceived unfavorably. Leave behind all your personal problems once you are on the externship site's property. For some people, this intention must be given thought well in advance. Most of us have various types of personal problems and pressures to deal with constantly: children, relationships, finances, and so on. Many people you will work with also have their share of issues, but they keep their jobs by showing up with the intention to do one thing: their job. If your personal life is not going well, make a complete success out of your externship! If all else is failing, make this your time to shine and improve professionally; deal with your personal problems at another time. Do not let your issues get in the way of reporting to your site daily and on time. You should acquire this habit before you enter the workforce; practicing it seriously during the externship is imperative.

The following constitutes the components of this detrimental perception:

- *The detrimental perception:* "I have so many problems to deal with, and I am so stressed. Spending a whole day at an externship just adds to it all. I cannot cope."
- *Signs of the detrimental attitude:* Distraction from working and learning, not acting professionally due to lack of focus and concentration.

- *The realization:* "The externship is short term, and it will benefit my professional growth to suppress the stress of other life issues while at the site so that I can learn and succeed and demonstrate to others that I am fully capable of professional-level work."
- *The good perception:* "This is easy enough. I simply need to shift my focus during the externship hours. I can and will present myself pleasantly and professionally. I can deal with my problems later."
- *Signs of a good attitude:* Ability to focus on work, a calm and pleasant demeanor, others (patients and staff) feel confident and comfortable with your work.

Detrimental Perception #5: "Something's always wrong."

If you tend to complain, now is the time to recognize that complaining is taboo in any professional office or facility. You can rid yourself of this tendency by setting the intention to improve this attitude.

If you complain often, chances are that you probably are not seeing enough of the good in life. Think about how it appears to staff members and patients when you complain. The staff at your externship site may assume that you do not appreciate the accommodation being made for you, and you may lose your position. Patients may feel uncomfortable if they hear complaining because they seek care with an expectation of competence and professionalism—a worker's complaining somehow undermines both of these.

If by nature you are a pessimist, intentionally shifting your focus to the positive aspects of life will require substantial effort on your part. It is to your benefit that your desire to succeed in your new career is likely to provide sufficient motivation for you to seriously put effort into this change. In fact, keeping your eye on the goal of succeeding in your career should be the underlying motivator for following all the advice provided in this guide, as well as other sources intended to assist you.

The following constitutes the components of this detrimental perception:

- *The detrimental perception:* "Why do bad things always happen to me? Nothing ever turns out right or good for me."
- *Signs of the detrimental attitude:* Frequent dissatisfaction, overreaction to minor inconveniences, recognizing and pointing out the faults of others, general appearance of unhappiness, customer service ability suffers.
- *The realization:* "Complaining will not help me in my professional endeavors. I can change this aspect of myself."
- *The good perception:* "Resolving not to complain, especially in a professional environment, raises my level of professionalism and effectiveness."
- *Signs of a good attitude:* Ease and a positive attitude in adapting to inconvenient situations, quick to seek solutions rather than complaining about the problem.

Attitudes that Promote Productivity and Success

By approaching your externship with the right attitude, you not only will be more helpful at your site but also will reap more benefits from the experience. Ways you can achieve this include the following:

- Caring for others
- Committing to serve
- Using good manners
- Showing enthusiasm

Caring for Others

Having chosen a division of allied health for your career, possessing an overall attitude of genuine caring toward people should be quite natural for you and your peers. You have chosen to be part of a team that is dedicated to caring for and serving patients and customers—hence the frequently heard terms *patient care* and *customer service,* aiming toward the goal of *patient and customer satisfaction.* This attitude should be present in all your professional encounters with staff and patients.

A patient or customer will become uncomfortable as soon as he or she does not feel that sense of caring coming from you (or any other staff member). Patients with problems are very sensitive to how they are treated in the medical establishment. They are even sensitive to this treatment in other situations, such as when discussing their issues over the phone with office staff, when visiting an outside facility for lab work, and when interacting with pharmacy staff about medications or insurance coverage. So put on a warm smile and use a gentle, concerned voice at all times, even when you may not be in the best mood. You will benefit too, by feeling the effects of positively impacting somebody else's day.

Committing to Serve

Make it your duty to serve, knowing that serving others with a positive and caring attitude is far reaching, for both you and those you serve. Leaders do not become leaders until they first serve others. Is your goal to advance into positions such as department head, office manager, or clinical manager? Or are you looking to be paid on the high end of the pay scale when you have more experience? If so, your service to others will guide you there in due time. Even when you achieve your goal of becoming a clinic, department, or office manager, or holding some other advanced position, you will be serving others even more, not just receiving more pay, prestige, and recognition.

The quality of service you provide to others (patients or staff) is determined significantly by your attitude. If your attitude is that everyone should cater to you (or serve your needs) and that you are supposed to be the center of attention, then your service to others will be minimal or nonexistent. If your attitude is that you chose your particular profession because you want to help others and you truly see the great value in doing so, then you will be among those who provide the most effective and most recognized service. Others in your working environment will quickly and easily grasp and remember this about you. Therefore, it is in your best interest to make the conscious decision—before you begin your externship—to show this attitude of friendly service.

Using Good Manners

It is very important that you *use good manners*. This seems elementary, perhaps something you learned in childhood and still value. However, a handful of adults and even highly educated people in the working world have not mastered the general rules of polite social conduct. Perhaps they work in professions where these skills are unnecessary, but in patient care and customer service the use of good manners is essential to demonstrate concern and respect for others. Good manners are the foundation of excellent customer service, and they reassure patients that they are well cared for and respected by those providing their health services.

The patients with whom you interact will expect politeness and respect from you, and your superiors in the office will respect you more when they see you demonstrating this to them and others. The same applies when communicating by telephone, whether you are setting appointments, calling in prescriptions or lab work, scheduling a surgery, speaking with a patient or customer, or resolving issues with an insurance agent. Thus, saying "Please," "Thank you," "Excuse me," and so on is necessary at all times. If your normal, daily vocabulary does not already include these pleasantries, practice and train yourself to do so. Your mannerisms and demeanor represent you, as well as the entire office or facility in which you are working and your school or college.

Showing Enthusiasm

Enthusiasm is a positive attitude that will carry you far in achieving your goals. Are you enthusiastic about starting your career? Are you motivated to learn and accrue experience? Are you excited that you will have many opportunities to help people in need? And will those working with you and those you are serving be able to see this aspect of you in your day-to-day performance? Not only can you brighten the day of others through your enthusiasm for your work, but you also can help yourself to be perceived by others as a worker who is content and confident.

Enthusiasm can boost the overall quality of your work. Patient and customer satisfaction remain priorities throughout all areas of health care, and enthusiastic workers who help achieve this goal are sought after by all employers.

HIGHLIGHT: Tips from Professionals

"We encourage our staff and externs to remember that your attitude determines your altitude. Our patients' healing starts when they come through the door and are greeted by our front office staff, and it continues throughout the visit and beyond, through their full recovery. We contribute to this with a positive attitude. The extern must have an attitude to serve. Service is not a term to be used only at restaurants, retail stores, and in business transactions."

Ivan L. Fennel
Coordinator, Pediatrics Office,
Clinical Research, and Community Health Outreach

Developing Perceptions and Attitudes at the Externship Site

You should seriously consider the preceding discussion of perceptions and attitudes before the externship begins. This section touches on those perceptions you might possibly develop once you have begun to take notice of the behaviors of other staff members during your externship. It is not intended to generalize and make assumptions about staff ahead of time but, rather, to raise general awareness.

The following scenarios are simply examples. These types of concerns do not present themselves in all externships. You may find that they assist you as you consider perceptions and attitudes at your externship site.

1. You are in a different position than those working around you at the site. You are "the student" or "the apprentice," not an employee who has been with the organization for five years. If an employee is demonstrating practices that are unprofessional or commonly discouraged while at work (talking on a cell phone, Web surfing, paying personal bills online, gossiping, and so on), take it upon yourself to have the sense *not* to exhibit that behavior. Just because you perceive that you are in a relaxed or nonchalant environment, as a student-extern you cannot assume any attitude or action that you observe, such as minimizing your effort because others do so. You must always draw professional boundaries for yourself and abide by them.

2. You may perceive that employees around you are talking about you behind your back. Although this is possible, do not retaliate with any type of negative attitude or action. If you can ignore it and concentrate only on your work, do so. If it bothers you and interferes with your ability to work or concentrate, speak to the manager or supervisor and, if appropriate, to your school's externship coordinator or liaison for advice.

   In this scenario, it is important to avoid wrongly accusing others simply because you have "a feeling" that they have acted in this way. Remember your position at the site as an extern: Do not exhibit any negative attitude or reaction that will put you in a bad position.

3. You notice after your first week or two that the general tendency among some people you are working with is to be caught up in "office politics." When you observe this type of drama, do not become involved, even if you feel that some individual(s) are attempting to get you involved. If given any opportunity to respond to this—don't. If you are asked for your opinion or to get involved in any way in such situations, simply and politely reply that you wish not to be involved due to your student status. Remember: Your professionalism counts toward your externship grade.

Give your attention immediately to any negative perceptions you realize you are developing. You do not want to develop any attitude that might cause you further problems. If you cannot check any negative perceptions you are developing on your own, speak with your school externship coordinator or liaison about the issue. Many times, simply discussing the scenario and listening to another's insight will help clear your vision and restore appropriate perceptions.

CONCLUSION

The attitude and perception considerations presented in this chapter are major contributors to successful externships. To maintain a positive attitude, focus on the positive aspects of life and, especially, on your commitment to succeeding in your career. Be a critic of your own strengths and weaknesses, and adjust your outlook accordingly. Your attitudes and perceptions greatly influence how you work and how professional you are. During your externship, be positive, appreciative, respectful, and willing to learn from your mentors.

Self-Prep Questions

1. Evaluate yourself. What attitude traits do you possess that will afford you a positive externship experience? What are some areas you think you should improve on prior to your externship?

_____

_____

_____

_____

_____

_____

_____

_____

_____

_____

2. If you were interviewing an extern to work with your medical office team, what attitudes would you seek in that person?

_____

_____

_____

_____

_____

_____

_____

_____

_____

_____

3. In previous positions or jobs you have held, what attitudes of your peers, co-workers, or managers that made them respectable and recognized workers do you recall?

_____

_____

_____

_____

_____

_____

_____

_____

_____

Role-Play Scenario

This scenario requires three individuals:

- *The extern,* who can be any type of allied health worker; simply adjust the role and content as needed
- *The customer or patient* who encounters this extern.
- *The supervisor* who oversees the extern and is the point of contact for the school's externship coordinator

The three individuals perform two short scenarios to reflect opposing ends of the attitude spectrum. The extern will decide whether to first act out the positive or the negative attitude. The direction the scenario takes will be based on how the staff person acts.

Open the scene with initial contact being made between the customer or patient and the extern. For example, if the extern is an MA, the scene could start with the MA calling the patient from the waiting area to the patient room. For another example, if the extern is a front office, billing, or pharmacy tech extern, the patient or customer could walk up to the desk to discuss a question or issue.

The extern should portray traits to create the negative attitude and the positive attitude, in two separate scenes. Participants should try not to overact and simply to play out what realistic attitudes can show, both positive and negative.

The third individual (the extern's supervisor) sees and hears the encounter between the customer or patient and the extern and then speaks to the extern concerning the attitude he or she portrayed in the encounter. These could be words of encouragement or reprimand, depending on which attitude scenario took place.

1. What are some realistic positive and negative attitudes that can be portrayed by the extern? Give at least three examples of each.

_____

_____

_____

_____

_____

_____

_____

_____

_____

_____

2. In each of the opposing scenarios, how would the extern's attitudes affect his or her ability to perform basic job duties well and to serve the patient or customer effectively?

_____

_____

_____

_____

_____

_____

_____

_____

_____

_____

_____

3. In each of the opposing scenarios, how would the extern's attitude affect the patient or customer?

_____

_____

_____

_____

_____

_____

_____

_____

_____

_____

4. In each of the opposing scenarios, what are the various ways the extern could expect the supervisor to handle the attitudes portrayed?

_____

_____

_____

_____

_____

_____

_____

_____

_____

_____

5. How can these attitudes affect the success and grade for the student's externship?

_____

_____

_____

_____

_____

_____

_____

_____

_____

6. How can the opposing attitudes affect the chances of the extern becoming employed through the externship or being referred for employment to another facility?

_____

_____

_____

_____

_____

_____

_____

_____

_____

_____

Readiness Checklist

_____ I recognize how my perceptions in certain areas directly influence my attitudes.

_____ I understand the likely pitfalls of possessing detrimental attitudes during my externship.

_____ I understand how the right attitudes can influence my overall success.

_____ I have identified any personal perceptions I possess that may become problematic.

_____ I have considered ways to overcome problematic perceptions for my externship term.

_____ I understand how my attitudes can affect the patients or customers I will serve.

_____ I know that I have the willpower to leave behind any personal issues or problems while at my externship site.

_____ I understand that I am still a student and am subject to the procedures and techniques recommended or required at my site.

_____ I can follow all required procedures and techniques with a positive attitude.

_____ I recognize the necessity of using good manners in the patient care and customer service settings.

chapter five

Etiquette and Professional Manners

Introduction

This chapter highlights the importance of using professional manners and avoiding unprofessional ones. Manners, and the lack thereof, say much about a person and can communicate both favorable and unfavorable characteristics. Several aspects of etiquette are well worth the attention of all allied health students entering the health care industry. Once identified, each point of etiquette is described in light of how it communicates various messages at the externship site. This discussion also demonstrates how correcting these tendencies can contribute to professional development while you avoid behavior-related pitfalls during the externship. The chapter concludes with Self-Prep Questions, a Role-Play Scenario, and a Readiness Checklist.

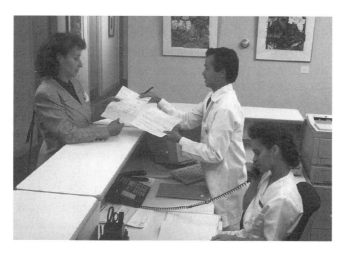

It is important to practice professional etiquette when assisting patients in person and on the phone, as well as when working as part of a team.

Chapter Objectives

- Identify the general meaning of the term *etiquette.*
- Identify the importance of appropriate etiquette in the medical externship.
- Identify at least three aspects of yourself that your posture can communicate.
- Name at least six additional manners that affect how others view you professionally.
- Explain the appropriate way(s) to deal with each of those six additional manners.
- Name at least four distracting behaviors that affect your professional demeanor.
- Explain at least one possible solution for each of those four distracting behaviors.

The Significance of Etiquette

Etiquette generally refers to the various manners and behaviors prescribed by and observed in social life. How do you carry yourself? How do you portray your work ethic? How can others see that you are committed to your work and concerned for your patients' and customers' welfare? These traits are all categorized within the context of your personal etiquette. Your etiquette speaks to others about you in many ways: how you work, whether you genuinely care, whether you are a committed worker, and so on. While you can show utmost respect for others and professionalism through your personal set of manners, it is crucial to recognize which manners, habits, and gestures are not acceptable in any professional setting, even while you are a student. Every person has his or her own unique set of manners that includes positive and negative (or unfavorable or unprofessional) aspects, and sometimes socially unacceptable behaviors are perceived as acceptable by the people who do them. Many people, even many who are highly educated or have a long history of successful work experience, still may benefit from tweaking their manners a bit to optimize their professional demeanor.

Students have been dismissed from their externship sites for behaving in an unacceptable manner, as well as for their attitude issues. Thus this entire chapter is devoted to the single topic of etiquette. Both acceptable and unacceptable manners are discussed. Self-presentation through posture, verbal manners, and professional language is analyzed, and basic tips on behavior are included.

Several particular aspects of your character say much about you, your confidence, your abilities, and your interests. For example, I worked with a student who was dismissed from two different sites for the same reasons. She had no problems arriving on time or doing as she was instructed, but her unprofessional demeanor and etiquette said more about her professional qualities than the two externship site managers were willing to tolerate. In this case, the main issues were not smiling (appearing grumpy), waiting to be told what to do (not taking initiative), slouching when sitting, leaning when standing, chewing gum, and showing an overall disinterest in learning. This combination communicated to both site managers that this student was not motivated, did not care about the staff or patients, and did not appear to have the potential to be a productive worker. Both site managers in this case indicated that this style simply does not work in a health care setting.

In summary, even if your skills and techniques are superb in the classroom, be aware of the more personal aspects that matter during the externship just as much as your technical competencies. In addition, it is important to pay attention to etiquette as you are preparing for job interviews; it determines much of the interviewer's first impression of you.

Etiquette for Allied Health Externs and Professionals

Several aspects of etiquette that will be important to focus on in your externship include the following:

- Posture
- Verbal manners
- Word Choice
- Avoiding distracting behaviors

Posture

Your posture says much about you. It reflects your confidence level and your attitude, as well as your interest in what is happening around you. If you slouch in chairs or lean frequently on desks and countertops, do you think the people around you will perceive you as confident and an effective or productive worker? Actually, those nearby will wonder what is wrong with you and may even think you are experiencing physical discomfort or pain. Patients will think this, too, which has important implications. Patients need to feel that they are being cared for by a high-quality and confident health care team, not by people who drag themselves around and twiddle their thumbs or who appear not to know what is going on. Patients and customers are more comfortable and satisfied with staff members who show interest, demonstrate care, and carry themselves professionally.

A poor or negative attitude often can lead a person to slouch, and anyone who slouches tends to repel people, especially if this posture is a chronic habit. Typically, this posture also reflects boredom, unproductiveness, and even lack of a work ethic.

A correlation exists between attitude and posture. Thus, changing one's posture comes easier to those who make a conscious decision to change the underlying perceptions and attitudes that originally led to slouching and leaning. (To review the importance of attitudes and perceptions, see Chapter Four.)

Disinterest in performing your everyday duties and learning as you work can easily convince others, including facility managers and physicians, that you may not be truly committed to your chosen career field. As a student-extern, demonstrating a lack of interest in your externship will not serve you well when it comes to your evaluation by the site manager or the opportunity to initiate professional contacts and relationships to jump-start your career. It is very important to assess your behaviors to ensure that you actually are communicating what you want to about yourself during the externship.

Verbal Manners

The level of professionalism you display with your verbal manners and associated tactics also affects how others view you professionally. These manners & tactics include how you speak to others, your listening skills, your ability to apologize, how you address conflicts and generally how you treat others. Consider the following specifics:

- Using manners as a mechanism of showing a favorable attitude was discussed in Chapter Four. The use of good manners should become natural for professional people hoping to be successful. It shows consideration and respect for other staff members and customers and patients.

- Speaking like a professional practitioner is another direct indicator of how professional you are in your field. This skill involves understanding and applying vocabulary pertaining to your specialty and avoiding the use of unprofessional fillers, such as "Um," "Uh," and "like" while communicating. (See the next section for examples of casual and improper phrases and their professional translations.) Keep a medical terminology book or medical dictionary handy so that you can easily check your use of professional medical terms. Your work team and patients form a more respectful perception of and confidence in you when you speak professionally.

- During the communication process, it is of utmost importance to steer clear of any tendency to interrupt when someone else is speaking. This tendency is sometimes irresistible, such as when you are convinced that the message being communicated merits correcting.

- Correcting or adding to somebody else's words or comments must done tactfully. Never correct a team member or engage in a confrontation in the presence of a patient or customer.

- It is a known fact that not a single person is perfect, so when the time comes that you make a mistake or handle something incorrectly, admit your fault and apologize. Also, state your intention not to make the same mistake again and, if possible, thank the person who pointed out your error. We tend to despise people who constantly correct us, but these corrections and what we learn from them build us professionally.

- When addressing conflicts, the best approach is to address them as situation-related rather than person-related. In other words, focus on the problem's aspects and seeking a solution rather than on anyone's faults and communicating these opinions to others. Engaging in the latter is a sign of immaturity and lack of professionalism. Also, addressing conflict from this viewpoint (situation-related) helps to reduce or eliminate further interpersonal issues due to the issue at hand.

- A reliable and relevant rule of thumb, often referred to as "the golden rule," is to treat others the way you wish to be treated. This means extending courteousness, forgiveness, encouragement, empowerment, compliments, recognition, and the like to others at the appropriate times. Aren't these what you hope others will extend to you?

Word Choice

It is important to employ grammatically proper, professional, and polite language in any professional setting, especially in allied health professions. Would you like to be acknowledged and respected as a professional? If so, your wording and tone of voice are as important as the array of other factors noted. Table 5-1 provides a short list of selected example phrases, along with the appropriate way to say the same thing in a professional environment. You will see that a few of these focus on the matter of tone, whereas others address proper English language usage. As others phrases come to mind, perhaps you

TABLE 5-1 Word Choice

Unprofessional Wording and Phrase	The Professional Alternative
What?/Huh?	Pardon? Excuse me?
Yah.	Yes.
Nah.	No.
What's up?	How are you?
What do you need?	How may I help you?
You ain't got … ?	Do you not have … ?
I ain't …	I do not …
I don't understand anything you just said.	Please clarify what you mean.
We don't got none.	We don't have any.

will recognize them and be able to think quickly of the more professionally acceptable wording and tone.

Avoiding Distracting Behaviors

Some distracting behaviors and conditions should be avoided while in the professional environment. The following delineates a few that are important, along with some recommendations.

- In a medical facility, pharmacy, hospital, or billing office, and especially during the externship, gum chewing should never occur. In fact, the office rules for staff likely include a written policy against it. It is offensive to some staff, customers, and patients, and the act of chewing gum does not fit the image of a clean, sanitary medical or professional environment.

  It is important not to have bad breath when working in close contact with others, but this can be achieved though proper dental care and should not be gum-dependent. A thorough brush, floss, and rinse are appropriate before work. Breath mints after snacks and lunch also are useful. Some foods, particularly sulfurous foods such as garlic, cabbage, and onions always should be avoided before working around others, as the sulfur compound in such foods causes bad breath.

- At times other than during a formal break, snack items should be consumed where designated and out of the sight of patients or customers. Food, wrappers, snack bags, soda cans, and the like diminish the image of a neat and sanitary medical environment. On occasions when a snack or tray of food is provided in the break area, you should demonstrate appropriate etiquette by taking a reasonable or small amount of food, even if you are very hungry. Be considerate of others who may come along after you for their portions. The best behavior is to wait until the regular employees have had their chance to take what they would like before you, the extern, partake of the lunch or snack. This is simply the courteous and respectful way to act in this situation. In addition, be sure to clean up after yourself after consuming food or drink on site.

- Another very important point to consider is that a practitioner who works in very close proximity to patients and customers should never smell like cigarette smoke while on duty; this is highly offensive to some staff members and patients. This particular odor also works against the goal of a clean, sanitary working environment.

- Do not appear tired. If excessive fatigue is an issue on any given day, it is important to find ways to cope other than showing such obvious signs as constantly yawning or resting your head in any way. Be sure you allow yourself enough nighttime sleep, as you will likely work full days during the externship.

While at your site, if necessary, ask to take a brief break, go outside, and take a three- to five-minute medium-paced walk in partial sunlight to reenergize. Consuming fruit and other types of healthy snacks during the day (rather than chips and cookies) also helps maintain your energy level.

- All phones and other portable devices, such as MP3 players and pagers, should be turned off or completely silenced while active at the externship site. These devices should not be visible to other staff or to patients and customers. This includes using the silent features of modern, advanced cell phones, such as Web surfing, e-mailing, and text messaging, even during a brief period of downtime at the site. Trying to squeeze in these electronic activities while on the job is highly unprofessional, and if perceived as a habit by the site supervisor, this may be another potential reason for dismissal from the site permanently. It may be acceptable to use these devices when officially "off the clock," or on break time, or it might not be allowed on site at all. Make sure you are in full understanding of the rules at your site concerning this issue. In any case, one definite rule of thumb is not to engage in these activities in the presence or viewing area of patients or customers.

- Regarding computer use at the externship site, it should not be assumed that because you have been placed at a computer station to complete certain tasks that it is okay to use the Internet for any personal reasons or to play computer games. This includes checking personal e-mail, paying bills, shopping, searching music and video downloads, and so on. Many computers have built-in games that become habitual for some people when no immediate task is at hand. These games must be avoided as well, especially when, as an extern, you are attempting to make your best impression on the professionals training you.

During the externship, it is important to give your best effort in all areas. Consider what personal adjustments are necessary, and plan ahead to be successful. The preceding list cites some of the most common areas of concern for student-externs to consider prior to the externship.

HIGHLIGHT: Tips from Professionals

"When at the site you need to speak as a professional. Come to work in clean scrubs, and having taken appropriate measures to maintain personal hygiene like showering and brushing hair and teeth. If the office has a casual day, be sure to dress appropriately."

Natasha Smith,
Medical Assistant, Electrophysiology Department, Multi-Facility Cardiology Practice

CONCLUSION

These aspects of etiquette are significant as you enter the allied health industry. The more personal contact and communication you have with patients, customers, and other health care professionals, the more important your manners become. The best way to ensure a good start is to visualize yourself in the setting, working with patients or customers and to zoom in to the impressions of you as their service or care provider that those patients and customers might develop. Think carefully about what areas you may need to improve prior to beginning your externship so that you do not have any etiquette issues interfering with your professional performance.

Self-Prep Questions

1. Name at least five behaviors or manners that are unacceptable.

   _____

   _____

   _____

   _____

   _____

   _____

   _____

   _____

   _____

2. What aspects of etiquette do you feel you should improve for your externship?

   _____

   _____

   _____

   _____

   _____

   _____

_____

_____

_____

_____

3. What are your etiquette strengths? How do you think these will promote you as a professional in your allied health specialty?

_____

_____

_____

_____

_____

_____

_____

_____

_____

_____

Role-Play Scenario

This scenario requires four to ten individuals, depending on class size (more if feasible). The scenario is an office party for a physician's birthday. The office is usually closed daily for the lunch hour, which is when the party is being held in the facility's break room. Set up a table with either snacks or a full lunch for the celebration. One to three students can be designated as the externs, while the others participating in the scenario are the employees. The group performing should act out the office party scene, focusing on proper etiquette but at the same time carrying on with normal eating, conversation, and interaction with others. The audience should have paper and pen readily available during the scene to critique observable etiquette and to present these details to the acting group at the end of the scene. Look for positive and negative etiquette aspects to note among all participants.

1. Make two lists, recording proper etiquette observations in one and "needs improvement" etiquette observations in the other.

_____

_____

_____

_____

_____

_____

_____

_____

_____

_____

2. Were any differences noted between the manners of the externs and those of the employees? If not, should there have been any?

_____

_____

_____

_____

_____

_____

_____

3. In a constructive manner, give your advice to the actors on how they can improve their etiquette. Reinforce the positive aspects you noticed.

_____

_____

_____

_____

_____

_____

_____

_____

_____

_____

_____

Readiness Checklist

_____ I understand the overall picture of how my manners or etiquette in the professional setting contribute to my professional demeanor.

_____ I have considered and recognize any changes I should make in my typical posture or demeanor.

_____ I understand the possible consequences of not appearing to have a positive attitude, confidence, and a noticeable interest in my field.

_____ I have considered ways in which I can improve my verbal manners.

_____ I have gauged my level of appropriate wording in general professional conversation and am aware of any challenges I need to overcome.

_____ I recognize the major distracting behaviors, and I have thought of ways to overcome those which may apply to me.

chapter six

Developing Professional Relationships

Introduction

This chapter presents the basic concepts of professional relationship development to keep in mind during the externship. This will likely be your first real-world experience in the position for which you have been training. Although much more framework exists for fully developing professional relationships, this chapter is tailored to prepare allied health students for the most preliminary of these considerations for the externship phase. The chapter concludes with Self-Prep Questions, a Role-Play Scenario, and a Readiness Checklist.

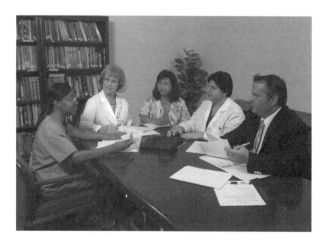

Teamwork, communication, and other aspects of interpersonal relationships contribute to the professional success of the extern and medical office staff members.

Chapter Objectives

- Identify five sets of skills that contribute to the development of professional relationships during the externship.
- Describe the interdependence that exists between members of the health care team.
- Identify specific ways to initiate and develop healthy interpersonal relationships.
- Identify five examples of poor communication tactics.
- List three types of communication.
- List two key factors that help complete the communication process.
- Briefly describe what is meant by the terms *verbal, nonverbal,* and *written communication.*
- List at least twelve effective communication tips to practice during the externship.
- Identify seven underlying causes of interpersonal conflict.
- Describe the meaning of conflict resolution and its benefits when handled successfully.
- Describe how to handle a personality clash in the workplace.

Building Professional Relationships

Your success as a professional depends greatly on your ability to effectively interact with other professionals. This involves fulfilling your role within the patient care team and avoiding or resolving difficult situations, such as personality conflicts that can affect your work. You should practice a specific set of skills in this area, including learning to be an effective team member, building healthy interpersonal relationships, utilizing effective communication skills, resolving any interpersonal conflicts, and respecting the differences in personalities among your peers. During your externship, tune in frequently to these aspects of professional relationships that define the working environment.

Functioning as a Team Member

By the beginning of your externship, you should realize that you are going to be part of a team. Although you may perceive yourself as an independent worker, it is important to realize the interdependence that exists among the various functional areas and departments of your externship site, in that each staff member relies on the correct functioning of and the receipt of correct information from all other staff members. This includes all clinical and administrative staff. If you are a clinical extern, your work as an MA, phlebotomist, X-ray technician, and such will provide important information for patient management and all treatment prescribed by the doctor, PA, or nurse practitioner.

After the appropriate clinical staff members visit with the patient, complete specific tasks, and document them in the patient chart, then the staff members working with medical records, insurance billing, referrals, prescription and lab order phone calls, legal issues, and such use the clinical staff's notes to complete the patient's visit and lay the groundwork for the entire cycle of care. All staff members are important contributors to the overall operation of the office or facility, including janitors, maintenance personnel, information technology (IT) professionals, and any other behind-the-scenes laborers, and you should acknowledge this by your interaction with others working on the same team.

Building Interpersonal Relationships

Building good interpersonal relationships as early as possible during your externship will help you significantly. You can initiate the development of such relationships by being willing to learn from and help others, by demonstrating courteousness, and by using effective communication skills. Many of the proactive measures you can take in this area are the active forms of the ideal attitudes presented in Chapter Four. For example, think back to the brief discussions presented on the positive attitude traits of pleasant service to others, appreciativeness, genuine caring, and persistent use of good manners. These coincide with learning from and helping others, as well as being courteous. Give a thank-you when someone reminds you where to find a piece of equipment. Lend a helping hand to a team member who might be behind schedule in his or her tasks. Also be helpful when interacting with patients and customers.

Communicating Effectively

Entire textbooks are devoted to the subject of effective communication. This text presents a few basic points that you should remember specifically for your externship, such as how communicating *effectively* influences your professional relationships. If you can achieve that skill, you will be in a position to say what you mean and to be interpreted by your listener or receiver as you intended. This enables you to avoid the consequences of poor communication, which can stall your learning and advancement in your field.

Among the numerous poor communication tactics you should avoid are blaming others, not thinking before you speak, talking too much, giving unsolicited and maybe even unwanted advice, and bragging, all of which will lead to undesirable results. Fortunately, all poor communication can be avoided with determination and practice.

The major types of communication are verbal, nonverbal, and written. Listening and feedback complete the effective communication process, and your capacity to listen effectively influences your overall communication effectiveness. Appropriate and meaningful feedback—a response you provide to others or that others provide you—is effective only when active listening is practiced.

Your actions, tone of voice, body language and gestures all fall into the category of nonverbal communication. The words, statements, questions, and commands you actually speak all fall into the category of verbal communication. The way you express yourself in writing (wording, grammar, and spelling) falls into the category of written communication.

Others can learn much about you through the way you communicate. In addition, as an active participant in the communication process, you should be able to accurately comprehend and interpret the feedback you are given by others. Recall the interdependency of the health care team described previously in this chapter, and imagine how effective communication is required for proper team functioning with minimal communication-based breakdowns or mistakes.

The following subsections contain tips that are highly applicable during the allied health externship for each component area of communication, and they are applicable to your communication with other staff members, as well as with your patients and customers. If you feel you need more tips on the art of effective communication, seek additional resources from one of your instructors or a professional within the career services department at your college or school. Many resources are available on this topic.

Verbal Communication   The words you speak should be clear and easy to understand. Speak using complete sentences. If you are working in a noisy environment, speak louder, but do not shout. The same applies when speaking to patients or customers over the telephone. Since you will be working in an environment where patient information must remain confidential, you must practice caution in how you communicate certain information and to whom it is communicated.

Nonverbal Communication   Your posture, eye contact, facial expressions, tone of voice, and overall professional demeanor contribute to the messages you communicate daily. Employ the following brief tips concerning these aspects of nonverbal cues:

- *Posture.* You should always try to maintain an upright posture (as opposed to slouching or rolling your shoulders down and forward). Recall the brief discussion concerning posture in Chapter Five on the topic of etiquette.
- *Eye contact.* Make eye contact with anyone with whom you are communicating. Avoiding eye contact makes others feel unsure about your confidence in what you are doing or saying. Also, it is simply not polite to avoid making eye contact. Add a smiling face to your eye contact.
- *Tone of voice.* Be sure that your voice conveys friendliness and not frustration. Work inevitably becomes frustrating at times, but it makes no sense to pass on this frustration to other workers and patients or customers. Falling into this trap creates friction in your work environment and may prompt customers or patients to complain.
- *Overall professional demeanor.* Consider your overall professional presentation as you communicate with others. Do you feel that others with whom you are communicating will perceive you as professional based on your appearance, gestures, and movements? And will they be able to clearly understand your communicated message in the midst of your unique mix of nonverbal cues?

Use these factors in positive ways to improve your customer service ability and to demonstrate professionalism. Patients and customers can read your body language and are more comfortable with their encounters with allied health staff when they can interpret that you are a sincere, caring, and helpful medical assistant, office staff member, billing representative, pharmacy technician, and so on. On the flip side, it is important and to your advantage to be able to interpret nonverbal cues from others, whether coworkers, patients, or customers.

Written Communication   Since most of your written communication will be patient information, it is extremely important to express the information accurately in writing. In patient charts, be sure to write the appropriate information in the proper section. Be certain that all words, numbers, and medical abbreviations are clearly legible, and use proper grammar, spelling, and punctuation. If you record the patient's chief complaint, for example, write clearly so that other team members (MAs, nurses, physicians, etc.) tending to the same patients will be correctly informed about the patient's explanation of symptoms or reason for the visit. For insurance, billing, and referral purposes, this supporting information must be accurate and easy to follow from the patient chart.

The same applies when working with electronic records. Consider all the possible parties within the health care system that may access a certain patient's health care information electronically. This information must be correctly entered with no errors. Excellent documentation practices are extremely important in any health care facility.

Listening   Pay attention, and make it a habit. Focus on the message being delivered to you by the spoken or written words of the communicator. Tune in to the nonverbal aspects of any message. Your feedback to the communicator cannot be fully effective until you have understood his or her original message. Ask for clarification if you do not fully comprehend the message, either what has been said or written to you. When interviewing or conversing with patients and customers, be sure you fully understand their complaints, descriptions of symptoms, questions about treatment options, questions about medications, and inquiries about their medical records or billing statements.

Feedback   Do you provide appropriate feedback to those who initiate communication with you? Listening is the key to the ability to provide proper feedback. Feedback should be relevant and timely. Your feedback may be needed immediately or later. Provide it at the appropriate time.

Practice diligence when providing feedback to patients and customers. You must stay within your legal scope of practice when communicating and providing feedback to them.

Issues of Conflict and Conflict Resolution

All students hope for a pleasant externship experience. Occasionally, however, some students experience interpersonal conflict with another or others at their site. We are all human, so it is not surprising that these issues arise, even if you are the most likable or delightful person.

Generally speaking, conflict is inevitable in the workplace at times. Personality clashes, differing values and perceptions, differing expectations and goals, ineffective communication, and competitiveness are all underlying causes of it. Most people see conflict as only bad; however, it also enables those who work through it diligently to reach resolution and experience personal and professional growth. The keys to a positive outcome are to recognize the onset of conflict before it causes anybody to compromise the effectiveness of their work and to find a way to resolve the interpersonal issue at hand. This is often referred to as *conflict resolution.*

If you experience any interpersonal conflict while at your site, seek advice or help immediately. Do not be quick to verbalize questionable or negative thoughts about others, especially while at your site. Instead, contact your externship coordinator and faculty regarding the issue. Be honest with the details of your personal perception of the problem, and consider any advice offered by your externship coordinator or career services staff. Depending on the situation, the externship coordinator may meet or speak with the site supervisor to discuss the issue and decide on an effective resolution.

Sometimes, the perception of one or more individuals is what causes an interpersonal problem. If this affects you during your externship, take a proactive role in attempting to resolve the problem. Alternatively you may ask "Couldn't I just

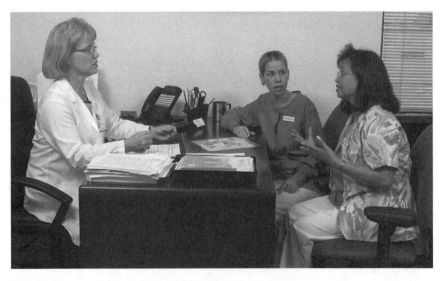

Effectively resolving conflict requires cooperation and teamwork.

be placed at a different externship site?" The answer given to my students is "No" until we all have attempted to reach a resolution.

A resolution is usually possible if all parties choose to cooperate. If you run away from the issues, you forego a chance to gain experience that may be useful later in your career, and the same type of situation is likely to arise again.

If it arises, interpersonal conflict can be the most challenging aspect of the externship. Working through it and overcoming it successfully will be a significant professional feat.

Overcoming Personality Clashes

You should expect that most people possess at least one personality aspect that you are not exactly going to like. You probably have friends and family who help you realize this. The important point is to respect everyone's differing personalities. If a quarrel with a friend or family member results from these differences, you typically have a good chance of reconciliation.

At your externship site, when you realize people's personality imperfections and conceive your own opinions about them, do not let those opinions get in the way of your reasons for being at that facility or office. Do not let such personal irritations hinder your professionalism either. When others "get on your nerves," the best action you can take is to move, if possible, to a different area to do your work. Another option, which will take some mental effort on your part, is to focus on your reason for being where you are and achieving your goals of learning and excelling in your externship. Maintain the mindset that you really don't have time and effort to waste on others' irritating habits.

If the situation or annoyance becomes personal in any way or interferes with your performance, you may need to speak to your externship coordinator/instructor and the site supervisor overseeing your work. On the other hand, remember that some of the people you are expected to work with may have opinions about *your* personality. Overlook personal annoyances and accomplish your goal of learning your specialty. Be realistic about the working world, expect that people will irritate you from time to time, and be empowered to overcome it.

HIGHLIGHT: Tips from Professionals

"Externs are 'guests' of the site, and therefore should not involve themselves with office politics. Work ethic is also important. If there is any downtime in the extern's work, the extern should ask the manager what else can be done to assist the others working. Whenever issues or problems arise, aim to minimize your complaints and think 'solutions.'"

Denise Wenger,
Office Manager, OB & GYN Group Practice

C O N C L U S I O N

In general, during the first few days of your externship, look for ways you can be an asset to the team. Appreciate everyone's role in helping you learn, and make it a habit to lend a helping hand to others when you see the need. If along the way you are affected by any personal conflicts, ask for advice and seek to resolve them. When people's personalities or habits irritate you, do not take it personally; continue performing your work as a genuine professional. Remembering and practicing these tactics will contribute to your overall level of professionalism.

Self-Prep Questions

1. Explain your role as an MA, administrative assistant, phlebotomist, X-ray tech, and so on in patient care. What will be your primary responsibilities? In what ways will you function interdependently with other professionals within the patient care team? (How will you depend on them and how will they depend on you?)

_____

_____

_____

_____

_____

_____

_____

_____

2. Recall the three major ways in which you communicate to others. Critique your own personal communication skills in these three areas, and identify the areas you may need to improve before your externship.

_____

_____

_____

_____

_____
_____
_____
_____
_____
_____

3. Briefly explain how listening and feedback are associated with effective communication.

_____
_____
_____
_____
_____
_____
_____
_____

4. What actions would you take, and in what order, if you were to become involved in some type of interpersonal conflict while at your site?

_____
_____
_____
_____
_____
_____
_____
_____
_____

Role-Play Scenario

Three individuals are needed for this scenario. The extern has been given some tasks to complete by the facility or office manager. One of the regular employees at the site is instructed by the manager to supervise the extern in completing these particular tasks for the remainder of the workday. This employee is normally the one who is working in the same area with the extern, but today he or she has been assigned this supervisory role, and the manager has just recently mentioned to both the extern and employee that this employee will be given the responsibility to supervise the extern for the second half of his or her externship.

Once the manager has instructed the extern in the set of tasks to be performed and has given responsibility to the employee to oversee the correct functioning of the extern, the extern begins to work diligently. The employee immediately lets this "power trip" go to his or her head. Although the extern is performing satisfactorily, the employee is constantly looking or listening (whichever applies, or both) for ways to input his or her opinion every chance possible and to find things to correct. The employee falls behind in his or her own work because of focusing on the extern's work and looking for problems. Finally, the extern is fed up with this and approaches the office manager with the issue. The office manager must then propose a solution.

1. How should the extern deal with the situation while still working in effort to finish the tasks on time?

_____

_____

_____

_____

_____

_____

_____

_____

_____

_____

_____

2. How long is long enough for the extern to attempt working under these circumstances before he or she approaches the manager with the issue?

_____

_____

_____

_____

_____

_____

_____

_____

3. How should the extern communicate this complaint to the manager about the employee-supervisor assigned to oversee his or her work? Write out or verbally state specifically how the extern should voice the complaint.

_____

_____

_____

_____

_____

_____

_____

_____

_____

4. What are some possible solutions the facility manager could propose?

_____

_____

_____

_____

_____

_____

_____

_____

_____

_____

_____

✓ Readiness Checklist

_____ I understand the nature of my profession in that I am always functioning as part of a team: I depend on the work of others and others depend on my work.

_____ I understand how to initiate healthy interpersonal relationships and that doing so boosts my level of professionalism.

_____ I realize that poor communication tactics have negative consequences. I have identified my tendencies in this area and will practice avoiding them for the sake of my success.

_____ I understand the importance of all three modes of communication in my career field.

_____ I realize that my skill in listening is essential to my overall communication effectiveness.

_____ I realize the various aspects of people that may lead to interpersonal conflict in the workplace.

_____ I understand the importance of seeking a resolution to interpersonal conflict, and I understand that during the externship it is important to seek help and advice from my faculty and site manager if a situation arises.

_____ I understand that people's personalities and habits may not be the style I prefer. In such situations, it is best not to let these aspects hinder my professional work in any way.

_____ I understand that effective interpersonal skills are extremely valuable during my externship, as well as in my future work.

_____ I understand how effective interpersonal skills contribute to my professional success.

chapter seven

Fulfilling the "Student" Role During the Externship

Introduction

This chapter addresses the basic actions to take during your externship for a successful experience. It describes how to be an active student-learner by being fully engaged in your work and taking initiative in your learning, while maintaining good student status. The chapter concludes with Self-Prep Questions, a Role-Play Scenario, and a Readiness Checklist.

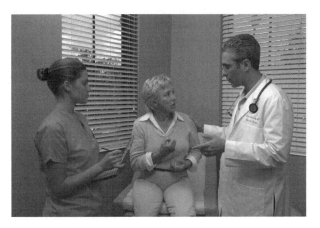

Fully engaging in the externship requires proactive learning. This includes listening, asking appropriate questions, and taking notes.

Chapter Objectives

- Explain the importance of fully engaging in your externship.
- Identify three benefits of fully engaging in the externship experience.
- Identify six examples of how to fully engage in your work at the externship site.
- Identify three drawbacks of not fully engaging in the externship experience.
- List six questions that will determine whether an extern is fully engaged in the externship.
- Name two ways in which an extern must be responsible to the supervising externship faculty or coordinator.
- Name at least five types of information that should be recorded in your daily externship notes or journal.

Fulfilling Your Responsibilities

To some students, the words *externship* and *internship* infer not being in school. Although physically you will not be on your school's campus, your externship site will become your temporary place of learning. Participation is mandatory, attendance is accounted for daily, and the accumulation of your efforts and performance will earn you your final grade, just like any other course you have completed. Many students are motivated to begin this phase; a few tend to see it as a time to slack and, therefore, do not take their responsibilities seriously.

This is the trade-off: You are expected to become fully engaged in your profession and apply all you have learned in the classroom while temporarily moving away from the type of learning that involves book work, classroom assignments, and exams. Thus, it is imperative that you perceive this phase as the most important part of your training. If you are thinking of slacking during your externship, or you have not established a serious mind-set concerning it, you risk losing control of your success, at least for the immediate future. Consider this seriously, keeping in mind that this is your first opportunity to earn a good reputation for yourself in your new career field.

Engaging In and Benefiting From Your Externship

Fully engaging daily in your work is a necessity; priceless benefits result from doing so. Remember: Nothing compares to the real-world portion of your training. Most disciplines of allied health are considered hands-on, intimate professions, and one benefit of full engagement in your practicum is perfecting or fine-tuning the technical skills you learned in the classroom.

No matter what your specialty is, daily practice of various tasks is essential for development of your practical skills. It is what you will be employed to do soon, so use this time to become more comfortable and more efficient in your techniques. For example, an MA externship includes such technical skills as taking vitals and blood pressure, giving injections, performing EKGs and urine analyses, drawing blood, documenting or charting, and scheduling appointments.

Another aspect of full engagement is realizing the scope of what it means to work as part of a professional team (see Chapter Six). Reading about team dynamics is a helpful start, but the actual experience is a form of learning that you are more likely to retain. You will have the opportunity to observe the levels of interdependence that exist among allied health, nursing, physician, administrative, and business staff members.

The facility staff at your site will notice whether or not you are engaging in learning and applying yourself, and this can work for or against you, depending on your level of engagement. Their observations will definitely matter for your externship evaluation and grade, and they could influence the start of your career. For example, staff at your site may be evaluating you discreetly for possible future employment, or they may be doing so for another office that may need to hire additional staff. You never know who is watching you or when. If you are fully engaged in your externship, you will definitely begin your career with a good rapport in some corner of the industry. This can help you tremendously in the future.

Following is a brief recap of the benefits of fully engaging in your work at the externship site:

- Fine-tuning your technical skills
- Experiencing working as part of a professional health care team
- Earning a good or excellent externship grade
- Developing good rapport with your site for professional reference in the industry

How to Engage in Your Work

To gain the most and best experience and knowledge, as well as to show your enthusiasm for the allied health profession, it is important to fully engage in your externship. This may be done in a variety of ways:

- Ask questions
- Take notes or maintain a journal
- Be present
- Solicit feedback
- Offer your help
- Take initiative and assume responsibility

Ask Questions You are a student, and the staff working with you will expect that you have questions or uncertainties every now and then—and more often in the first few days of your externship—as you become familiar with the setup and daily operations at the site. Asking questions benefits you in ways other than just clarifying your uncertainty. For example, it shows the staff and site supervisor that you are interested in getting things done right and that you are respectful of adhering to the preferences of the staff, doctors, and so on.

Take Notes or Maintain a Journal   Good students take notes in class, and although you are not in a classroom during this phase, it is important that you treat the externship as another class—that is, you should try to absorb as much new information and insight into your profession as possible. You might be required by your specific program of study to maintain a journal or compile daily notes for a similar assignment. Documenting your experiences, new skills and techniques learned, and other general professional experiences in a journal or notebook is useful for personal reference or for any later project or writing assignment having to do with your externship. It also demonstrates to the site staff and supervisor that you value their input and methods of training and that you are a responsible trainee.

Be Present   With or without acceptable reason for it, some extern students find themselves slacking off when it comes to site attendance. Yet the importance of attendance cannot be emphasized enough since you will not learn or progress without regular attendance and fulfillment of your commitment. Poor attendance also irritates and inconveniences site supervisors and trainers because it makes it impossible for them to complete their own plan for your training. This is such a serious matter that your absence at scheduled times may result in you being dismissed permanently from the site. *Take your schedule seriously.*

Solicit Feedback   Don't wait for your final evaluation at the end of the externship to gauge your progress. Make it a point to ask your supervising staff trainer or manager each week for input on your performance. Ask what areas they think you need to improve, whether your efficiency in getting tasks done is up to par, and how they would assess your professional development. Those training you will consider it very responsible and professional of you to ask these questions. Plus, you will have ongoing (for the duration of your externship) feedback with opportunities to improve as you progress through your training.

Offer Your Help   As many professional site supervisors would state, "Don't just sit there!" During a slow time at your externship site (if this actually happens), do not be reactive—be proactive. If the time comes when you have run out of things to do or you have completed your assigned tasks early, ask what else you can do to help. This is another way to get involved and learn about other areas of health care functioning that will be helpful to you in expanding your understanding of the whole health care process, thereby adding to your professional development.

Take Initiative and Assume Responsibility   Make yourself the type of worker who is always active. Adopt the attitude that you have an important job to perform and people to serve. When problems or issues arise, think about possible solutions and ask others for assistance rather than leaving the issue alone simply because you are not an official employee. Help set up and clean up. If customers or patients are waiting to be greeted at the check-in desk, and no other employees are available at the moment, greet the customer or patient and state that the appropriate staff person will be available shortly. Adopting habits like these help you quickly develop into a productive and desirable worker.

The Problem of Disengagement

In significant ways, not engaging in your work daily has its drawbacks. First, if you are overly disengaged, your site may dismiss you permanently since staff trainers tend to view having such an extern as a waste of time.

Second, community and regionally associated medical facility managers and administrators tend to know each other through professional organizations and affiliations, and they converse often. The last thing you should want is for your name to be associated with the label *"Caution!"* within your local professional community. The health care community is eager to praise those who work hard and go the extra mile, but recognition is also widespread of individuals who regularly are unproductive or have attendance or personal issues at work.

Third, your personal disengagement while you are at your externship site is detrimental to your learning. If you are not active daily in taking on the challenges presented and learning from others, you are jeopardizing your own opportunity to gain everything mentioned in the previous paragraphs. Essentially, it would be a waste of time to go through the externship without the will to learn and grow professionally. So, do the opposite: Engage in your learning.

The following briefly recaps the drawbacks of not fully engaging in your work at the externship site:

- Probable dismissal from the site
- Beginning your career without the rapport you otherwise could have gained, and possibly creating your own negative vibe that can spread through parts of the local health care community
- Wasting your time and the valuable opportunity to learn more for your own professional growth

How to Be Fully Engaged

If you are reading this in advance of your externship, use the following questions to prepare to be fully engaged in this learning experience. If you have already begun your externship, use the following questions to determine if you are fully engaged in it:

- Do you attend your site as scheduled and arrive on time daily?
- Do you arrive prepared?

HIGHLIGHT: Tips from Professionals

"Treat the externship like a professional job. Extend common courtesy to patients and staff. Punctuality is also important; call the office when unable to show up for scheduled hours. Don't just sit there doing nothing during slow times – find something to do."

Julia Baez, R.N.
Office Manager, Internal Medicine Practice

• Do you have a positive and helpful attitude every day?
• Do you ask appropriate questions to enhance your learning?
• Do you take notes or keep a journal?
• Do you attempt to learn about areas of office functioning other than those in which you typically work?

Acting Responsibly

To ensure that you are being a responsible student and fulfilling all of your externship requirements, you should follow these steps:

• Maintain communication with your school.
• Maintain an academic or learning mindset.
• Maintain proper procedure for absences and tardiness.

Maintaining Contact with Your School

Aside from the effort you put forth at your site, you have other responsibilities as a student. You must maintain active communication with your externship coordinator and any other faculty or staff from your school that are involved in your externship or program completion (financial aid office, registrar and student account offices, career services, etc.). You should note what contact is expected of you prior to beginning your externship. Your main contact obviously will be with your externship coordinator or supervising faculty member. You will be responsible for providing a verifiable record daily or weekly of your hours attended. If the proper information is not provided by you, you probably will not receive any credit for your attendance. Do not expect the externship site supervisor to be responsible for submitting your hours for you unless the arrangement between your school and the site manager requires this. If your assigned method of submitting hours is via fax, follow up the fax with a phone call to verify that it has been received. Take initiative in these areas to maintain favorable student status with your college.

Maintaining an Academic Mindset

Since you are technically still a student while an extern, you should envision yourself for the entire externship in student mode, maintaining an academic mindset. Realize early that this time will provide a significant learning experience. Just as you take notes in the classroom, you should take notes daily while on the externship. Keeping a daily journal may or may not be required by your academic program. Some programs require you to submit a final report on your externship experience for a grade.

Whichever requirements apply to you, optimize your learning experience by recording a few notes daily about your experiences. A hidden benefit of doing this is that you can prepare for questions that may be asked of you during future employment interviews by reviewing these notes to vividly recall your experiences. Besides simply noting what happened and how to perform new procedures, make notes of what types of teamwork came into play, how you learned to communicate more effectively, and what strengths and weaknesses you discovered about yourself. Maximize your insights as much as possible for the sake of your personal and professional development.

CONCLUSION

The externship is a new and completely different learning phase for you, but it is important to fully engage in learning while still a student and to equip yourself with all the knowledge you will need concerning your school's contact, attendance, and graduation processes. You will be off campus, and for some students, it's very difficult time-wise to get back to campus once in the field for the practical phase. Be sure to speak to your immediate supervising faculty members to be sure that your expectations and vision are targeted correctly.

Self-Prep Questions

1. How do you plan to fully engage in your externship experience? What aspects of your technical skills and professionalism are you seeking to exercise?

_____

_____

_____

_____

_____

_____

_____

_____

2. Do you know your school's protocol for submitting externship hours? How often are time records due? How are the hours verified? What is the penalty for not following this protocol?

_____

_____

_____

_____

_____

_____

_____

_____

_____

3. How are your school's attendance and tardiness policies applied to the externship?

_____

_____

_____

_____

_____

_____

_____

_____

Role-Play Scenario

Two to four individuals are needed for this scenario. The extern arrives at the office or facility as scheduled and finds that the office manager (no part to be played) will not be at the site today. The extern has already been on externship with this staff for 2 weeks. Create a scene showing how the extern can create a productive working day without the guidance of his or her usual site supervisor. (Other than the extern, the other individuals participating should be regular employees who work in surrounding areas at the site.)

1. What are the initial steps the extern can take when discovering his or her usual leader will not be available to assign and oversee tasks? (There are several options for appropriately handling this situation.)

_____

_____

_____

_____

_____

_____

_____

_____

_____

_____

_____

2. How can the extern devise a plan of action for the day?

_____

_____

_____

_____

_____

_____

_____

_____

_____

_____

3. Create a plan the extern can work from to achieve a productive work day.

_____

_____

_____

_____

_____

_____

_____

_____

_____

_____

_____

✓ Readiness Checklist

_____ I understand the significance of fully engaging in the externship.

_____ I understand the shift in my responsibilities in the change from classroom learning to off-campus learning.

_____ I am motivated to engage in and complete the externship.

_____ I recognize the benefits of fully engaging in the externship.

_____ I recognize the drawbacks of not fully engaging in the externship.

_____ I understand how to determine whether I am fully engaged in learning at my externship site.

_____ I am prepared to keep daily notes or a journal of my learning experiences during the externship.

_____ I know my school's written requirements (if applicable) for completion of the externship and how it will contribute to my grade.

_____ I understand that during the short-term externship, I should not experience any tardiness or absences, unless an emergency situation arises.

_____ I know my institution's policies and procedures for tardiness and absences, and I have considered the fact that I will have to compensate for any time missed.

chapter eight

Benefits of Successful Externship Completion

Introduction

In this chapter, you will gain insight into the personal and professional benefits that come with successfully completing the externship. This chapter motivates allied health student-externs to perform well in all aspects covered in previous chapters so that the maximum benefits available can be gained. These benefits include the fine-tuning of technical and people skills, documented practical experience in the new career field, new professional contacts and relationships, a beginning point for networking, at least one new professional reference, and possibly a job opportunity or direct link to one arising out of the externship. The chapter concludes with Self-Prep Questions, a Role-Play Scenario, and a Readiness Checklist.

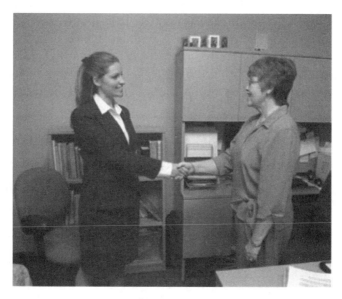

An appropriate place to initiate your professional network is with your externship site supervising staff members.

Chapter Objectives

- Explain the significance of the experience gained through the externship.
- Identify actions you can take to maximize the experience gained during your externship.
- Identify the factors surrounding the possibility of you becoming employed through the externship experience.
- Define networking, and explain how it can influence your career opportunities.
- Identify how to update your résumé with the details of your externship experience.
- Explain the importance of obtaining a professional reference from the manager or supervisor at the externship site.

Your Entrance into the Field of Health Care

This chapter revisits the idea presented in Chapter One that your externship is the *bridge* you must cross to advance from classroom work to the beginning of your new career. It is only after you complete the practical phase that you will be qualified with experience in an appropriate allied health setting. To emphasize the importance of the experience you will gain, it is typical that a medical office or other facility will prefer, or in some cases require, a certain amount of work experience in the field or your specialty as a condition of employment. Other preferences or qualifications, such as a specialty certification and proof of graduation from an approved program of study, may be required as well. However, these qualifications are on many occasions co-requisites to the level of experience required. In other words, your diploma or degree is not necessarily going to be seen by the health care community as a substitute for experience, so it is extremely important that you take full advantage of all aspects of experience offered to you by your externship. Your connection to your chosen career field begins in the externship; it could very well be your opportunity to get your "foot in the door" in various ways, which is what this chapter discusses.

HIGHLIGHT: Tips from Professionals

"Experience is a key component of the externship process. It gives the extern an opportunity and confidence to assure potential employers that they are ready to provide quality, reliable, efficient care to patients in a manner that will assist the practice to operate smoothly and to administer patient care effectively. Learning is an ongoing process in the medical field. The externship process reinforces the principles and practices learned in the academic setting. A great externship experience can be the difference in you being told how much you will earn and being asked what it will take to get you to be part of the team."

Ivan L. Fennel
Coordinator, Pediatrics Practice, Clinical Research and Community Health Outreach

The Big Benefits

The following are just some of the benefits you will receive from successfully completing the externship:

- Refining your skills
- Starting your career
- Networking
- Field experience
- References and letters of recommendation

Refining Your Skills

First, as emphasized previously, take full advantage of the opportunity to put your skills to work in the real-life setting of your externship site. Fine-tune your skills and your ability to be versatile by being useful in many areas of the facility throughout the workday. Learn about as many areas as possible, even those that are not what you prefer to do most. For example, you may be an MA who enjoys working one on one with patients in clinical procedures such as EKG and phlebotomy, but your externship should be balanced to include the full spectrum of clinical and administrative tasks. Remember that you are still in training and will eventually have the opportunity to seek out employment more focused on your preferred area of practice. The broader your experience is in the externship, the greater the number of experiential skills you can claim later as professional experience. Not only should you learn as many techniques and practices as possible, but you also should pay attention each day to other areas, such as customer service, patient interaction, and team interaction. This type of learning is beneficial to you and may even help you to answer certain soft skills–type questions as you interview for employment in the near future.

Career Launch Opportunities

Assuming you have performed according to all the rules and expectations of your externship, the opportunity exists to become employed from the externship or to obtain a strong referral for employment to another facility or office. If you develop a good, working relationship with the team at your externship site, and the office manager is in need of an extra employee, you may be a favored candidate since you will have trained with the team already. Obviously considering you for employment would imply that all your skills are exceptional according to this team of professionals: your interactions with patients, your technical skills, and your reliability.

You have little control when it comes to being offered a job with your externship site. Some offices engaged in training new externs are not in a growth phase and do not have the space or resources to add staff. However, the facility manager at your site may know that a branch location or an affiliated or neighboring office is in need of new MAs, phlebotomists, billing representatives, administrative staff, pharmacy technicians, and so on. What an opportunity that presents—and without the work of looking for vacant positions. Such opportunity has presented itself to many students who have put forth their best effort during externship, and a similar opportunity may arise for you.

Industry Networking

During your externship, you definitely will have the opportunity to network with staff. This refers to you talking to various individuals and marketing yourself by building relationships and trust in your career field. Of course, you will begin your networking activities at your externship site. As you gain experience and meet people from various parts of the industry, you will develop a unique network of individuals through whom you can seek opportunities. You also can inform those with whom you network of opportunities that may be suitable for them. The more people you know and with whom you have working relationships, the more opportunities you will have access to while developing your career.

An easy place to begin your networking efforts, even before your externship, is at your school. Your instructors, your externship coordinator, and especially your school's career services or job placement department may be able to recommend a few local starting points. Appropriate places to begin include, for example, on-campus career fairs and large-scale community- or citywide career events.

Field Experience

Once you have completed your externship, and before seeking interviewing opportunities, you should add the specifics of your externship experience to your professional résumé. This will enhance your marketability for your initial job search. Remember that your résumé should provide an accurate, professional, and positive image of you since employers usually will see this document prior to meeting you and learning about you. Refer to Chapter Eleven for résumé-building tips.

The externship is very useful when you want to include experience in the field on your résumé. List the name of the site, the beginning and end dates of your time there, and the total number of hours you completed for the externship. Then list the duties in which you were trained and those you performed. Also include all the skills that you applied. Use proper terminology and spelling to describe everything. This section of the résumé is especially important to graduates who are entering the various allied health specialties for the first time. In addition, if you have volunteer experience in a related setting, be sure to include a full description, as this type of experience is also impressive to many professionals.

Professional Reference and Letter of Recommendation

Many employers seek professional references or letters of recommendation from job candidates. Through your externship, you have the opportunity to acquire a letter of recommendation from your site supervisor and to ask that person if he or she will permit you to use his or her name as a professional reference. Do this completely at your discretion, but if you have worked well with the team members at your site and have maintained good, positive working relationships throughout your externship, it is to your professional advantage to seize this opportunity.

Final Touches

On the last day of your externship, do not leave without handing your résumé with correct contact information to the site supervisor. If you were responsible for providing your résumé prior to the externship, simply ask your supervisor if he or she would like another copy that includes the externship experience you just completed. If your mentors at the externship site become aware of a job opening elsewhere for which they may refer you, you definitely will want them to have your most recent qualifications and contact information within reach.

If within a few months of your graduation you sit for and pass one of the credentialing or certification exams in your field, notify your externship site supervisor of this by offering—in person—an appropriately updated résumé with this information. Each time you increase your professional qualifications, provide all your key networking acquaintances with the details, starting with your externship site supervisor(s).

As a courtesy to those who have accommodated you at the externship site, it is highly recommended that you send a thank-you note or card to express your appreciation for their roles in your learning. Recognize them for taking time from their schedules to help you, and mention how valuable the experience was for your personal and professional growth. See Figure 8-1 for an example of a brief thank-you note.

May 31, 20XX

Dear Patricia Davis and staff,

I would like to send you my sincere thanks for accommodating me in my externship and for all your efforts in my professional training. The opportunities you have provided to benefit my learning are invaluable, and I am greatly appreciative to have been able to work and gain experience with all the staff.

Sincerely,

(Your Name)

Figure 8-1. Example of a thank-you note.

CONCLUSION

As is apparent, you can reap numerous benefits from the effort you pour into your externship. While still practicing the skills you learned in the classroom, you must have the mindset that this externship is really your first point of entry into your field and that many benefits are to be gained. Take advantage of the possibilities presented, and tailor them to suit your needs in gaining a professional edge.

Self-Prep Questions

1. Recall the benefits available to you through the externship experience.

_____

_____

_____

_____

_____

_____

_____

_____

_____

_____

2. What are some specific approaches to effective networking?

_____

_____

_____

_____

_____

_____

_____

_____

_____

_____

_____

3. Check the newspaper or Internet employment ads for your geographical area and your field of expertise. What variations are cited for the preferred experience or education level?

_____

_____

_____

_____

_____

_____

_____

_____

_____

Role-Play Scenario

Two individuals are needed for this scenario. Imagine you are an extern who has completed your externship hours; today was your last day with this site's staff and manager. *The scenario:* Your supervisor has planned a meeting time with you before you leave the site to review your performance and how you have progressed since the beginning of your externship. (For general purposes of this scenario, the supervisor gives positive feedback and is impressed with your performance.) After this session, you initiate a brief discussion with the supervisor in effort to begin professional networking for your upcoming job search. Prepare ahead of time how you will approach this opportunity and what specific assistance you will request from your externship supervisor in these search efforts.

1. What assistance will you request from your site supervisor? Be sure you are professional in making your requests.

_____

_____

_____

_____

_____

_____

_____

_____

_____

_____

2. What plan will you establish for maintaining periodic contact with your site supervisor?

_____

_____

_____

_____

_____

_____

_____

_____

_____

_____

✓ Readiness Checklist

_____ I recognize that the externship is a significant link between my classroom education and my professional career.

_____ I understand that my documented work experiences are important considerations to my potential employer(s).

_____ I realize the opportunity and value in fine-tuning my skills, as well as building cross-functional skills.

_____ I realize that my externship site is a valuable entity as it may likely become an important professional referral source or possibly a future place of employment.

_____ I understand that in order to expect a strong referral opportunity with the staff at my site, I must excel in applying my technical skills, interacting with patients and other staff members, and showing reliability.

_____ I understand that my externship site can be a valuable first resource in my professional networking efforts.

_____ I plan to add the details of my externship experience to my résumé promptly on completion of my externship.

_____ I understand the importance of updating my résumé, as well as updating my key networking contacts with this information, each time I enhance my professional qualifications.

chapter nine

Performance Evaluation and Your Grade

Introduction

This chapter summarizes the general areas in which most allied health externs are evaluated on completion of the externship. It presents straightforward explanations of the variations that are possible within evaluations, depending on which specialty of allied health you practice.

The areas of evaluation cover practical, clinical, and technical skills; administrative skills; and professional qualities. Beyond the evaluation given by the externship site's monitoring supervisor, a few other requirements may contribute

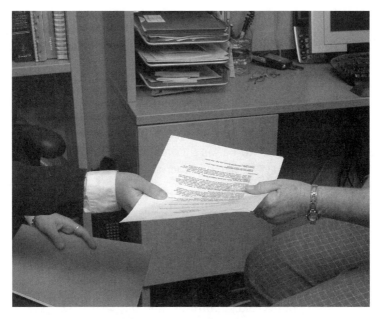

Your effort and performance determine the results of your externship evaluation.

to your final externship grade, such as a written report or other paperwork applicable to the practicum. The chapter concludes with Self-Prep Questions, a Role-Play Scenario, and a Readiness Checklist.

Chapter Objectives

- Understand the nature of the externship evaluation or grading process.
- Recognize the types of competencies included within each area of an externship evaluation: practical, clinical, and technical skills; administrative skills; and professional competencies.
- View samples of externship evaluation items for medical assisting and medical office administrative assisting.
- Identify several other possible requirements of the student-extern for the end-of-term grade.
- Understand the content recommended for other possible course requirements.
- Identify various grading categories encompassing the externship performance that can contribute to the final grade.

The Significance of Your Performance Evaluation

The overall goal of the practical phase of your education is to experience a set number of hours in a professional allied health setting in your specific area of training. However, it is important to remember that this phase is also a course requirement in which you will earn a grade. Your school normally maintains a syllabus or a guidelines document that defines the evaluation methods.

The way you are evaluated in your externship is substantially different from the classroom grading criteria to which you are accustomed. This is a time when you have the opportunity to be taught and evaluated by a qualified professional of your chosen industry—a person other than your regular faculty. By the final phase of your externship training, you should be looking for as much professional advice and constructive criticism as possible to help yourself prepare to enter the industry with confidence and reasonable expectations. While you should perform at your highest potential, do not become frantic because you are going to be evaluated. You will find that the evaluation helps you to recognize your strengths more clearly and to identify areas in which you need improvement or extra practice. If you take these points seriously, especially the ones identifying your weakest abilities, and do what is necessary to overcome them, you will be adding significantly to your professional development and value as an allied health professional.

The Basics of Evaluation

Various competencies for most allied health externship evaluations can be classified into three broad categories: practical, technical, or clinical skills; administrative skills; and professional competencies. If you are practicing an allied health specialty with more specific skill sets (other than medical assisting and medical administrative/office assisting), your evaluation will not include the range of skills applicable to MAs and MAAs, as illustrated in the following examples, but it will include the set of skills in which you have been trained. Also, externship skills and performance evaluations in some allied health programs can be divided into more specific categories or groups of competencies. If possible, at the beginning of your externship request from your instructor(s) a list of the evaluation competencies in which you will be assessed for your externship. Familiarizing yourself with the focal points of your evaluation will help you define your profession's job duties more clearly.

Medical Assisting Skills Evaluation

The following questions focus on competencies that are likely to be included in most MA student-extern evaluations. Generally, the evaluator will rate your abilities on a given scale or will answer questions about whether or not you demonstrate competency in each of the skills or techniques listed. Questioning yourself concerning these skills prior to your externship will help you notice areas in which you may need additional practice before beginning your externship. This is another proactive approach you can take for yourself to be better prepared for this training phase.

Professionalism, Career Development, and Readiness Competencies

- Do you show interest and intent to learn?
- Do you demonstrate critical thinking skills?
- Do you demonstrate attention to detail?
- Do you show empathy for all those you are serving?
- Do you follow professional ethical standards?
- Do you take initiative?
- Do you demonstrate flexibility or versatility?
- Do you adhere to the dress code?
- Do you have a clean and neat appearance?
- Do you use a systematic approach to problem solving?
- Do you demonstrate dependability (arriving to the site on time daily)?
- Do you show ability to organize work?
- Do you demonstrate effective time management skills?

- Do you work as a team player?
- Do you work independently?
- Do you complete tasks on time?
- Do you demonstrate a positive, cooperative attitude?

Administrative Competencies

- How competent are you in efficiently handling correspondence?
- How competent are you in filing charts and other records?
- How competent are you in using effective communication skills?
- How competent are you in using proper telephone etiquette?
- How competent are you in greeting patients courteously?
- How competent are you in operating a computer?

Medical Assistant (MA) Practical and Clinical Competencies

- How competent are you in preparing patients for routine exams?
- How competent are you in assisting the physician or other practitioner during exams?
- How competent are you in maintaining the physical environment of exam rooms?
- How competent are you in assisting with routine eye exams?
- How competent are you in utilizing medical and surgical asepsis?
- How competent are you in appropriately using personal protective equipment (PPE)?
- How competent are you in properly performing EKGs?
- How competent are you in properly performing venipuncture?
- How competent are you in explaining treatments and procedures to patients?
- How competent are you in applying knowledge of sterile fields?
- How competent are you in administering medications appropriately?
- How competent are you in obtaining and recording vital signs properly?
- How competent are you in obtaining and documenting patient history appropriately?
- How competent are you in accurately documenting physical exam measurements and results?
- How competent are you in applying medical terminology?
- How competent are you in collecting and testing urine samples appropriately?
- How competent are you in applying documentation skills?
- How competent are you in obtaining throat cultures?

- How competent are you in applying X-ray techniques and positioning? (If this is required of your profession, check state regulations for working with X-rays as requirements vary from state to state.)
- How competent are you in using lab slips properly?
- How competent are you in recognizing and practicing in accordance with HIPAA compliance standards?
- How competent are you in abiding by the legal and ethical standards of your practice?

Medical Administrative and Office Assisting Skills Evaluation

Another allied health discipline that covers a wide range of skills is medical administrative assisting. Students practicing in this area are evaluated in a number of competencies that includes the full spectrum of tasks normally performed by administrative and office assistants in a medical facility. While remaining focused on providing quality customer service to patients, such students are primarily focused on the business aspects of the medical facility, such as maintaining records and paperwork, handling office phone calls and reception, scheduling appointments, processing insurance and payments, billing and coding, and so on. The following questions address the practical skills evaluated for a medical administrative assisting externship. The professional and administrative skills listed in the preceding section are also applicable. Evaluations can instruct the evaluator to rate your abilities on a given scale or may ask whether or not you demonstrate competency in each of the skills or techniques listed.

 HIGHLIGHT: Tips from Professionals

"The training as a medical assistant encompasses many skills in the health care industry. The MA must view him- or herself as an asset to the clinical team since the skill set required covers both administrative and clinical responsibilities, thus providing a circle of continuity for the patient's visit. In addition, the MA utilizes basic employability skills, the three R's, decision making and problem solving, as well as team building to achieve a successful work experience. The three R's—reading, 'riting, and 'rithmetic—are some basic educational skills that enhance the student's marketability. Some examples of the areas where inadequacies in these may be reflected are in doing growth charts, calculating BMIs, spelling, and front desk skills."

Toni Moody, M.D.,
Pediatrician; Principal Investigator, Founder, and Executive Director of a community health organization

Medical Administrative Assistant (MAA) Practical Skills

- Do you effectively coordinate patient appointments and scheduling?
- Do you demonstrate proficiency in collection and verification of patient insurance information?
- Do you submit insurance claims accurately and on time?
- Do you process patient payments accurately?
- Do you monitor reimbursement by third-party payers?
- Do you document accurately?
- Do you properly and efficiently file charts?
- Do you follow appropriate standards in helping maintain patient records?
- Do you correctly understand and use medical terminology?
- Do you understand and apply office policies and procedures?
- Do you use professional phone skills?
- Do you use professional communication in all forms of written correspondence?
- Do you understand and properly use diagnostic codes?
- Do you understand and properly use procedure codes?
- Do you recognize and practice in accordance with HIPAA compliance standards?
- Do you abide by the legal and ethical standards of your practice?

Learning from Evaluation Results

You may be evaluated in a wide range of areas. Educational institutions do not use identical evaluation methods or forms, but a comprehensive MA evaluation will contain the preceding major areas, with more or less variety. Typically, the MA would be rated for each of these competencies. Also, you may notice that the items in the Professionalism, Career Development, and Readiness category are those that are emphasized in this text. They are all significant features of your hands-on training and indicators of your overall level of professionalism. It is possible to conquer all the challenges of practical skills and administrative skills, but without professional abilities and attributes it is nearly impossible for one to succeed or maintain a good job record in any part of the allied health field. If you feel you are weak in these skills, do not be discouraged. Deciding to improve yourself in the appropriate areas and following through on a planned course of action will help you to overcome any weaknesses and to develop your professional attributes. Depending on the feedback you receive from your evaluation, seek assistance immediately from your instructors in any technical skills needing improvement and from your school's externship coordinator/faculty or career services/job placement assistance department in any professional skills in which you need improvement.

It is possible to do the externship in a facility in which some of the listed clinical competencies are not applicable. For example, if the externship takes place in a cardiology office, obtaining a throat culture, performing routine eye exams, and testing urine would not be applicable skills that would be evaluated in that setting. Likewise, the utilization of surgical asepsis skills would not apply in a family practice or general pediatrics office in most cases. Many evaluation forms typically allow for a *not applicable* (N/A) rating for instances such as these.

Other Externship Completion Requirements

In addition to the practicum itself, many programs stipulate one or more other items that the student must complete. As noted in Chapter 7, two of the most common are a daily journal to be submitted on completion of the required hours or an end-of-externship written report. Another requirement that is oftentimes required is an externship site evaluation in which the student has the opportunity to provide his or her personal and professional opinion about the site in which he or she trained. Know ahead of time about these student responsibilities by checking the syllabus and communicating with your faculty/coordinator. More specifically, determine from your syllabus or asking your instructors how these various end-of-term assignments are evaluated and how they will ultimately contribute to your final grade.

Journal of the Externship Experience

In assignments involving a journal (see Chapter 7), be sure to provide meaningful insights in the comments you record. Journal assignments may require somewhat brief, daily input or a weekly (or longer) more detailed account of your experiences Unless you are given a specific format to follow, the most effective insight you document is what new information or techniques and practical skills you learned, along with a summary list of the actual duties you performed for the given day. To go the extra mile in this effort, you may briefly record your experiences and outcomes in the areas of working as a team player, how effective or ineffective communication affected any situations, and how you may have gone beyond your assigned duties to help another (or how someone else did this for you).

Projects and Written Reports

End-of-term projects or written reports are most easily composed by those students who maintain a journal of their externship experiences. At the same time, for relatively short externships, many of the experiences will remain memorable enough to prepare the project or report immediately on completion of the required hours. Unless provided with a specific format to follow in writing a report, the following are several categories in which your experiences can be grouped to help you organize the experiences and insight you intend to present:

Topic Categories for Written Projects or Reports

- Briefly describe the personnel structure, type of facility, and medical specialty or specialties practiced at the facility.
- List all the skills you applied during the externship.
- List new skills or techniques you learned that cross into other areas of the medical office or facility operations.
- Identify aspects of professionalism you were able to practice or enhance.
- Identify one or two instances in which conflict occurred within the team's functioning, and give your insight into the matter.
- Identify the most challenging aspect of your externship.
- Identify the greatest benefit that you believe you gained through your externship experience.

Student Evaluation of the Externship Experience

Many students are required to complete an evaluation of the externship site. This allows the student to give feedback from his or her point of view as to the helpfulness of the staff trainers, the appropriate exposure to various profession-specific situations and tasks, and the opportunity given to apply relevant procedures and techniques and operate equipment. It also provides helpful information to the program faculty of the school, and it ultimately provides a benchmark reference for each facility's capacity to train students in various areas.

Grading

The final externship grade is calculated based on the criteria provided to students in the respective externship syllabus. Numerous factors can be used to determine the course grade. The following are several categories—but not all that are possible—that can be evaluated and applied with a given weight toward the final grade:

- Professionalism
- Patient interaction and/or customer service
- Employee/team interaction
- Practical skills performance
- Written assignment(s)/journal/report
- Following instructions
- Time management
- Hours completed/attendance

CONCLUSION

The externship will be evaluated on your performance in many attributes of professionlism as well as on your skills performance and objective measures such as written assignments. The externship is your first opportunity to combine your best efforts in all areas of your prior training and to practice being a real allied health professional. Successful performance in all areas throughout the entire training phase will lead you to excel in the externship—and in the launch of your new career.

Self-Prep Questions

1. Identify the objectives/goal(s) of the externship according to the course description given in your college catalog and/or course syllabus.

_____

_____

_____

_____

_____

_____

_____

2. Identify the method of externship grade determination according to your course syllabus. (What categories are weighted together to determine your final grade?)

_____

_____

_____

_____

_____

_____

_____

_____

_____

Role-Play Scenario

Two individuals, or groups of two, are needed for this scenario. The purpose of this activity is to become familiar with the evaluation form that will be provided to your externship site supervisor and staff for feedback, as well as to understand how its results are formulated into a grade. One individual should act as the school's evaluating instructor/externship coordinator; the other should act as the student. The acting student is to attend a brief meeting with the externship coordinator to receive feedback given by the site supervisor with whom he or she has just finished the externship. The externship coordinator previously should have worked out the evaluation grade according to the school's scoring criteria. He or she discusses with the student the different skill sets evaluated and corresponding marks received and then explains how the evaluation grade has been calculated according to the syllabus.

1. According to your college/school's criteria, how are the scores classified and weighted to provide the final evaluation grade?

_____

_____

_____

_____

_____

_____

_____

_____

_____

_____

_____

_____

2. How does this evaluation grade fit into the overall determination of the final externship grade? What percentage of the grade does it comprise? What other requirements/grades will be weighted with this to determine the overall externship grade?

_____

_____

_____

_____

_____

_____

_____

_____

_____

_____

_____

Readiness Checklist

_____ I know the number of hours I am required to complete for my externship as stated in the course syllabus.

_____ I understand that a significant portion of my externship grade will be determined based on the evaluation of my performance as judged by my site supervisor(s).

_____ I have discussed with my instructor(s) the set of skills in which I will be evaluated by the site supervisor, or I have viewed a document showing these.

_____ I understand the distinctions among the general categories of practical skills, administrative skills, and professional competencies.

_____ I am aware of all other course requirements I must fulfill in addition to the completion of the required hours.

_____ I am prepared to excel in my externship!

chapter ten

Allied Health Externship: Case Studies

Introduction

This chapter presents nonfictional situations that have actually happened during student externships. The purpose of analyzing these cases is threefold: to reinforce the importance of the lessons presented previously in this text; to demonstrate the importance of true professionalism during the externship; and, of course, to help all current and future externs to avoid making the same mistakes. These scenarios reveal a wide range of areas in which the student-extern must be fully prepared to begin the practical phase of training in a professional health care facility, pharmacy, billing office, lab, or other appropriate agency related to the provision of health care. These cases reinforce many aspects of professionalism, as well as areas of practical skills readiness. Each case is followed by a few questions to guide the student in examining its key components.

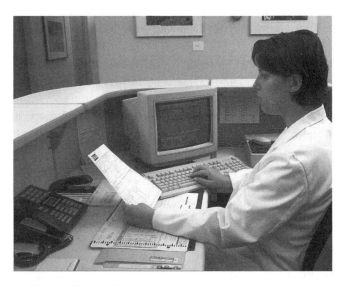

Professionalism and preparation are required of students participating in the externship.

Chapter Objectives

- Examine various real-life scenarios of student externship issues and dilemmas.
- Discuss the implications of the given situations.
- Provide possible solutions for improving the outcome of each case.

Case Studies

The following case studies are all nonfiction, but fictitious names are used to protect privacy. All externship requirements and expectations were given to all students when they entered the program of study, and these requirements are acknowledged by the students' own signatures required in externship paperwork packets. Specific requirements and instructions were given to students prior to the start of the externship, usually while students were in the final phase of coursework.

Case Study 1: A Delayed Externship

Tammie was scheduled to go on externship in May. She was an MA student. She had been out of school at least five months prior to the externship but had previously completed all coursework necessary. She re-enrolled in school so she could complete the externship and earn her diploma. When the time came for her to complete her pre-externship paperwork and to begin planning with the externship coordinator, she could not be contacted at the phone number on file with the school. She did not answer or respond to any of the many messages left for her in regard to the urgency of her contacting the faculty by phone or by physically visiting the campus.

A few weeks into the externship term, she finally notified the faculty that she was ready to begin externship. However, during the preceding weeks of no contact, she was dropped from the student body according to administrative policies. Obviously her externship had to be postponed again, and she was required to wait for the next term to begin.

Meanwhile, Tammie received all the necessary paperwork and instructions for the required physical exam and TB test. Although she had a few weeks to complete these tasks, when she contacted the college to begin the externship she still had not gone for a physical exam or TB test. Therefore, her reentry for the term was cancelled due to the lack of required documentation. *Externship simply cannot be initiated without completed paperwork.* Tammie waited again for the next term to begin. By that time, she had completed the health documentation and was finally set to begin the externship. All of this, beginning with the first re-enrollment attempt to complete the externship, spanned four months—just to *begin* the externship!

1. Give a brief analysis of the issues and problems involved in this case.

_____

_____

_____

_____

_____

_____

_____

_____

_____

_____

_____

_____

_____

2. Explain the measures the student should have taken and when in the context of this situation.

_____

_____

_____

_____

_____

_____

_____

_____

_____

_____

_____

_____

_____

Case Study 2: Attitudes and Impressions

Daniel was in the process of fulfilling his externship hours in an internal medicine office. His programs of study were health information technology and office administrative assisting. His site supervisors had established a methodology of training throughout all areas of the office pertinent to Daniel's educational training.

The first area of externship experience arranged was working with patient files, paperwork, appointments, and light correspondence. After the first two weeks of a part-time externship schedule, and having already missed two days of attendance, Daniel began to show the attitude that he was above and beyond this level of training, although he had never worked in a physician's office before. His idea was that he would go straight to the billing and coding area of the office, which actually was planned for the final phase of his externship by his site manager. As his "too good for this" attitude showed more each day, and as the professionals working with him took notice, the office manager finally contacted his college to inform the faculty of the attitude issues and that the office staff would no longer accommodate him. Therefore, this student suddenly was without an externship site.

The externship coordinator arranged a possible replacement site for Daniel, which required an externship interview. The interview time was agreed to by all parties four days in advance for 11:00 a.m. on the following Monday morning. On the day of the interview, Daniel showed up for the interview at 12:00 noon—and without a résumé. The site supervisor, who happened to be the owner of the company, conducted a brief interview with him. However, for obvious reasons the owner did not view him as a fit candidate for externship at that office. Therefore, Daniel was again without a site.

So far, one week had lapsed since he had earned any externship hours or credit. A few days later, Daniel was scheduled to meet with the office manager of a third possible site. He arrived on time with his résumé for this appointment, and after a brief interview he was accepted to begin externship the following week. (This delay is normal as many site managers need some advance notice to arrange to accommodate a student.) By the time Daniel was able to begin earning externship credit again, he was in severe danger of being dropped from his program due to nonattendance. Only through the persistence of the faculty and college administration were a few grace days allowed for him. The student completed the externship within a few weeks, but did so carrying on with habitual complaints and imperfect attendance due to personal issues.

1. Give a brief analysis of the issues and problems in this case.

_____

_____

_____

_____

_____

_____

_____

_____

_____

_____

_____

_____

_____

2. Describe what cooperation was needed from Daniel during his time at the first externship site. What benefits would have resulted from this? What differences in the outcome of his externship would have resulted?

_____

_____

_____

_____

_____

_____

_____

_____

_____

_____

_____

_____

3. State briefly the lessons that can be taken from this case.

_____

_____

_____

_____

_____

_____

_____

_____

_____

_____

_____

_____

_____

Case Study 3: No Show, No Site

Jaclyn was scheduled to begin her externship on Wednesday morning at 9:00 a.m. On Wednesday, the manager of the externship site called the externship coordinator to report that Jaclyn did not show up and had not contacted the staff. The externship coordinator then contacted the student to ask why she was not in attendance. Jaclyn's explanation was "I did not go to my site this morning because something I ate last night did not agree with me, and I have not been feeling well. Late at night I needed to take medicine so that I could sleep. I was supposed to be at my site at 9:00 a.m. today. What do I do?" The student and the externship coordinator both called the site, and fortunately the site manager was willing to issue a "grace" day in this situation and allowed Jaclyn to start on Thursday morning at 9:00 a.m. During this session, the student was reoriented by the manager concerning the importance of daily attendance and professionalism, which were reiterated by the college faculty as well.

The following Monday, the externship coordinator received another telephone call from the site manager with the report that Jaclyn again had not shown up or contacted the staff. This time the manager stated that this was the final chance and that the student would need to complete her externship at another site. The externship coordinator contacted Jaclyn regarding this incident, and she reported the following: "I'm so sorry I overslept. Nobody woke me up this morning. My cell phone alarm was set, but it was underneath my pillow and I didn't hear it." Jaclyn was then informed that she had lost her site assignment, that she would have to wait until another one could be arranged, and that she would need to participate in the site search as well to expedite the process. More than a week passed before she was able to resume her externship at another site.

1. Give a brief analysis of the problems and issues in this case.

_____

_____

_____

_____

_____

_____

_____

_____

_____

_____

_____

_____

_____

2. Suggest basic measures this student should have taken to prevent this unnecessary pitfall.

_____

_____

_____

_____

_____

_____

_____

_____

_____

_____

_____

_____

_____

_____

3. If you were the site manager in this case, what inferences about the student would you make concerning her neglect in contacting the office these two days?

_____

_____

_____

_____

_____

_____

_____

_____

_____

_____

_____

4. If you were a manager of a health care facility, would you refer this student to another facility or office for an employment interview? Think about how this pitfall will automatically give students a negative reputation professionally, as well as what losses to the student may result.

_____

_____

_____

_____

_____

_____

_____

_____

_____

_____

_____

Case Study 4: Confidentiality Breach

Samuel began externship in a medical office to train in administrative assisting and medical billing. In the beginning, his ratings were high from his supervisors. They usually gave positive feedback concerning his attitude, performance, and professionalism. Several weeks passed before his externship coordinator was surprised to receive a phone call that Samuel had crossed a major line, legally and ethically.

The report was given that an acquaintance of a close friend visited the office with his spouse for the spouse's appointment for psychiatric evaluation and consultation. Apparently, the student said "Hello, how are you doing?" to this acquaintance, just to be friendly. The specifics of what happened out of the office are not clearly known. However, the patient (spouse of the student's acquaintance) visited the office shortly thereafter to complain that an office worker had spread the word that she had consulted with a psychiatrist for whatever reason. The patient told her physician that she had received information from a friend regarding the news of her office visit. In summary, this private information had come back to her (the patient) through others whom she had never informed of this personal event. The information allegedly was initiated by Samuel, the extern, who was the only person in the office remotely acquainted with the couple.

Due to this incident, Samuel was no longer allowed to participate in the externship in this office. Not only did Samuel suffer consequences, but it also hurt future externs because the physicians and office manager made the decision that no externs would ever be allowed again in that role in their practice.

1. What violation was committed by this extern?

_____

_____

_____

_____

_____

_____

_____

_____

_____

_____

_____

_____

2. What are the possible consequences not mentioned in the case that could have arisen at a later time for Samuel?

_____

_____

_____

_____

_____

_____

_____

_____

_____

_____

_____

_____

3. What were the consequences to Samuel's college and fellow students?

_____

_____

_____

_____

_____

_____

_____

_____

_____

_____

_____

_____

Case Study 5: The "A" That Slipped Away

Brianna was challenged to meet the minimum hours required each week for her externship. However, she persevered throughout the externship phase and met the expectation in this area. On completion of her externship, she was required to submit several documents, including an evaluation by the site manager and several assignments regarding the externship experience. The following specific items were required and outlined in the externship syllabus as follows: evaluation by site (25 percent of final grade), student's evaluation of the site with short essay (25 percent of grade), journal of daily activities (25 percent of grade), and completion of all hours required (25 percent of grade).

Brianna's evaluation by the site was submitted on time, and her score provided by the site manager reflected excellence in all areas, including professional, administrative, and practical skills. Brianna opted to submit her journal weekly with her timesheets, so this requirement was fully met also. She completed the total hours in the time stipulated by the college, and so this requirement was fully met as well. Several days after the completion of her externship, the college faculty and externship coordinator were still awaiting submission of her evaluation of the site with essay documents to comprise the final 25 percent of her grade. Several more days went by with phone calls to the student attempted but resulting in the determination that her phone number was out of service. E-mail was used to reach her regarding this final assignment needed, but no response was provided by this means either. Finally, the grade was due for the externship term, and Brianna's final grade was calculated based on the items completed.

Her grade resulted in a C (75 percent) because she earned a zero for a component of the grade worth 25 percent. Even with a perfect evaluation by her site manager, her neglect in submitting the final assignment dropped her grade from a potential A (100 percent) to a C. This is a drastic difference between what the grade actually was and what it could have been.

1. What are the simple steps Brianna could have taken to prevent this major deduction from final grade for the externship?

_____

_____

_____

_____

_____

_____

_____

_____

_____

_____

_____

_____

_____

_____

2. Explain why understanding the syllabus guidelines for grading the externship is so important.

_____

_____

_____

_____

_____

_____

_____

_____

_____

_____

_____

_____

_____

_____

_____

_____

Case Study 6: Skills Revival

Michael was set to begin his medical assisting externship at a family practice facility. Before the externship, he responsibly submitted all the college-required paperwork on time. Also, he excelled in the skills evaluation required before his externship. He even was approved by his instructor while in the final phase of coursework to assist new students in learning how to read a blood pressure.

Michael began the externship with high expectations by his faculty due to his excellent performance throughout his courses. Within two weeks of beginning the externship, Michael's site supervisor notified the externship coordinator that Michael did not seem to be competent in his skills, specifically blood pressure reading, venipuncture, and injections. She also reported that Michael seemed exceedingly shy around the patients and staff. In addition, Michael did not take initiative to inquire about what he should be doing and for the most part was waiting for a staff member to give him step-by-step instructions on what task to complete next. The site supervisor stated that Michael did not seem like he had the ability to function on his own as an MA in an office or other facility. She also recommended that Michael return to the college for a brief review with the faculty before returning to the site. The site supervisor had good intentions in advising this as she did wish for Michael to perform well, demonstrate his competency, and become a qualified MA.

The staff at this office communicated what it thought would be the best route to improvement based on working with Michael. They hoped they would be able to truthfully provide good marks or ratings for his final evaluation.

Michael returned to her college and worked with several faculty members on various skills for a couple of days. After a complete hands-on skills evaluation, Michael was again deemed competent in all clinical skills applicable to medical assisting. After questioning Michael about specific aspects of how he was interacting and fitting in at his site, one instructor advised him in the area of taking initiative, smiling and appearing pleasant, being assertive rather than acting shy, being relaxed rather than nervous in his venipuncture and injection procedures, and taking charge of his role now that he had learned how the office functioned. (All these specifics are very relevant to how professionals at an externship site perceive the abilities and professionalism of student-externs.)

Michael returned to his college with these key points in mind. Several days after his return to the site, the site supervisor and other staff reported that Michael was performing much better, seemed more interested in his work, and had been communicating much more effectively with the patients and staff. Since he was taking more of a proactive role in his work, he was able to work more in the lab. He also had opportunities to prove his injection skills to another medical assistant, and he was then allowed to perform several venipuncture procedures with patients.

Michael also was proactive in requesting that another MA work with him on using the type of sphygmomanometer native to the facility's patient rooms. He proved his mastery of this skill as well. According to his evaluation by the site staff, Michael completed the externship with a good-to-excellent outcome.

1. What externship outcome was likely to have resulted if Michael did not take the advice from his instructor to be assertive, take initiative, and so on when he returned to the site?

   _____

   _____

   _____

   _____

   _____

   _____

   _____

   _____

   _____

   _____

2. Explain how a lack of initiative and assertiveness could send the message to a site supervisor or staff member that a student is not satisfactorily competent.

   _____

   _____

   _____

   _____

   _____

   _____

   _____

   _____

   _____

   _____

   _____

HIGHLIGHT: Tips from Professionals

"We have had a great many externs in our practice over the years. The first piece of advice before starting the externship is to practice your skills. We have had a number of (MA) externs who could not properly perform blood pressures or pulses. Personality is important, especially when dealing with the patients. I have had to remove a few externs due to their inability to communicate with patients.

Do not use your new externship site for free medical care; such needs should be met elsewhere. Punctuality and attendance are very important. Treat your externship like it was a paying job. Many times, I have had externs not show for their shift and not call. I feel this is also significant and shows how reliable—or unreliable—you are."

Paula Kennel,
Office Manager, Family Medicine Practice

chapter eleven

Beyond Externship: Beginning Your Job Search

Introduction

This chapter introduces the basic steps to be followed in the job search. It blends general expectations with various specialized aspects for allied health job searches. Student-externs should begin the preliminary steps of this phase during the externship, if possible, or immediately upon externship completion, unless further education or coursework is still to follow before program completion. The topics covered include becoming familiar with local job markets, writing résumés and cover letters, preparing for a successful interview, and following-up interviews with thank-you letters. To optimize the job search, it is highly recommended that, in conjunction with using this guide, you work closely with your career resource center on campus if available.

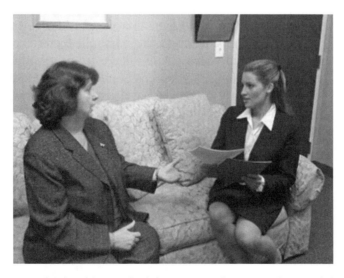

A professional image, both in person and on paper, is essential in successfully progressing through the job search, application, and interview processes.

Chapter Objectives

- Identify resources for becoming familiar with the local job market.
- Describe the goal of an effective résumé.
- Identify and compare the four basic résumé formats.
- Define *transferable skills* and give examples.
- Describe and identify an effective entry-level résumé.
- Identify specific allied health qualifications that should be included in the résumé.
- Describe appropriate formatting for building the résumé.
- Describe appropriate writing for building the résumé.
- Explain the overall goal of the cover letter.
- Describe how to accomplish the goal of the cover letter.
- Explain the importance of appropriate voice-mail messages and e-mail addresses for professional correspondence.
- Describe the proper attire and appearance for an interview.
- List the issues of etiquette to be followed for the interview process.
- Describe the goal and the main contents of the thank-you letter.

A Process with Many Steps

Multiple steps are involved in the job-seeking process, and you can put forth effort in many ways to improve your interviewing skills. The earliest search phase includes building your résumé and gaining a general idea of the job market in your geographic region. Consider going the extra mile by researching the companies or medical practices in which you are interested prior to the interview; this will prepare you to ask intelligent questions of interviewers. Other considerations include writing and submitting a catchy cover letter to submit with your résumé and then writing a sincere thank-you letter to all interviewers shortly after your interviews. Practicing professional etiquette and dressing appropriately for the interview are also important, as interviewers form their first impressions of you based on your actions and appearance.

All your efforts in these areas will prove significant as you strive to secure a position you desire. In general, taking a proactive approach to your job search will provide you with the best results.

Becoming Familiar with the Local Job Market

Gaining familiarity with the job market in your area is a process that requires time and diligent searching, beginning with the fact that employers advertise job openings in many ways. While it is quite easy to use various Internet job and career sites to find advertised positions, this will never provide an adequate picture of the available jobs in a given city or region. Also, Internet methods of collecting résumés are more likely than local resources to be limited to "collecting." Some companies do maintain their Internet postings simply to collect résumés without actually having an immediate need for employees. This is not meant to discourage anyone from searching within these Web sites. The job descriptions and salary information, if noted, provide useful information for all who seek employment. In addition to job sites on the Internet, refer to the listings of jobs by category in local newspapers. These sources are likely to contain postings by local organizations for positions that are somewhat immediate. Respond to ads for positions listed in local sources within a day or two of the posting. Check the same source as often as it is updated, and you will begin to gain familiarity with the demand for certain jobs within allied health, the minimum qualifications and experience required, and possibly the salary range, although some companies choose not to publicize their salary information.

Other approaches to job searching may require more time and effort. If you are interested in certain companies, hospitals, or health care systems, go directly to those organizations' Web sites. A link to "Jobs," "Employment," "Human Resources," or some other related page is usually accessible from the organization's home page and will lead you to a listing of available positions.

Various actions will then be required of you, the applicant. Many organizations have an online electronic application that prospective candidates must complete, and possibly a designated field in which you are to copy and paste or upload your résumé. Anytime a résumé is to be submitted online, be sure that the font is one of the basic types and that no graphics, word art, and such are present. It will be helpful to create and store a second résumé specifically for electronic submission, especially if your original résumé contains bullets or fonts that can become corrupted during electronic submission. When your application is submitted directly through a company's Web site, it is important to take time to complete the application in its entirety, emphasizing your marketable qualifications in the appropriate areas. Always proofread the electronic application before submission.

Other resources that may be available through your school or college are the on-campus career services, career resources, and job placement offices. The people working in these offices generally have a working knowledge of the latest job opportunities and areas of employment growth within the local communities, and they often offer students and graduates assistance with creating and updating their résumés, writing their cover letters and thank-you letters, and learning about successful interviewing. Most also have ongoing relationships with various employers, which can be very helpful to graduates of allied health programs.

Another great opportunity for students and graduates is to keep abreast of the schedule of various job fairs that take place within local and nearby communities. Information for these events can typically be found online at various job Web sites, on local TV news coverage, via radio commercials, and from career assistance offices. It is beneficial to attend these events even while still a student and to present yourself professionally: wear clothing appropriate for interviewing and carry a professional-looking organizer large enough to hold at least ten unfolded copies of your résumé. At these events, employers seek to collect résumés from job candidates and, sometimes, to perform on-the-spot interviewing and hiring. Perfect your interview techniques and other formalities, such as a firm handshake and professional introduction of yourself, by the time you attend this type of event so you can make a very positive first impression with potential employers.

Depending on the outcome of your externship experience and whether a good relationship was built with the site manager and staff, you can network with previous trainers and mentors about job openings in their facility or other facilities with which they are affiliated or acquainted. Provided that a very good to excellent externship experience took place, the staff from the site will likely be able and willing to give your name and a good recommendation to their peers. Try to maintain this level of relationship with your externship site staff for at least a few years. If this is feasible, always provide the staff at the site with a periodic update of your experience and increasing qualifications.

Whichever combination of these resources are used to begin the job search, you are advised to be as proactive as possible when researching the local job market. Those who take the approach that their school or college is responsible for their employment, even when job placement assistance is provided by the institution, lose many opportunities that they may otherwise discover for themselves by networking and using additional methods. The career assistance offices within schools are valuable resources, especially for students and graduates without experience in the job-seeking process; however, the services they provide should be accompanied by your own search efforts to maximize opportunities. Motivation is key in this process, and the motivating factor is that the amount of effort put forth in the job search will provide a proportional amount of opportunities for interviews and employment options.

The benefits gained by taking this approach are:

- You can see for yourself what the trends are in minimum qualifications
- You can recognize a group of effective key words relevant to the field in which you are seeking employment (useful in résumés and cover letters)
- You can use various resources to keep abreast of industry demands

Résumés

This section introduces three basic types of résumés, some valuable résumé tips, and sample résumés. The main concept to recognize in building an effective résumé is that it must paint a clear, realistic, and desirable picture of the professional *you*. It must reflect the totality of your accomplishments and professional experiences.

Essentially, your résumé is your application for an interview. Think of the moment when a potential employer is looking through a stack of twenty-five résumés, one of which is yours. How will you ensure that yours will stand out among the others? Those selected for interviews have presented the most appropriate, impressive, and easy-to-follow résumés.

Selecting the most appropriate résumé format conducive to your work history, experiences, and education will provide the best picture of you. Utilizing a style that is appealing will also tempt the reader to take a moment to peruse the content of your résumé. Organized headings with impressive, but not overdone, wording will also hold the reader's attention. While attempting to impress, it is important not to exaggerate content, wording, and design to the point where the résumé becomes gaudy, wordy, ambiguous, and difficult to follow.

The following sections will guide you through the basics of building a résumé.

Choosing an Appropriate Résumé Format

In building a résumé, you should consider certain aspects of your educational and work history prior to deciding which résumé format to follow. If you already have a résumé, use the following information to evaluate whether you have your personal work history presented optimally for your career goal. Any of several types of résumé can be utilized, and every individual should attempt to maximize his or her chances of obtaining an interview or becoming hired (or even of being accepted for the externship). The four main types of résumés are the chronological résumé, the functional résumé, the combination résumé, and the entry-level résumé.

The Chronological Résumé The chronological résumé presents the candidate's experiences in reverse-chronological order. The work experience is listed beginning with most recent and is identified by the position title for each entry. (Employers want to see *first* what you have been doing most recently in the workplace.) For each entry, the dates, or at least the month and year, are clearly shown, followed by the job title, company/employer name, job description, and accomplishments.

This type of résumé is best used by individuals who have a long, solid work history with minimal gaps between jobs. If a goal of the candidate is to demonstrate job stability, this is the optimal format. This type also accentuates position titles that are impressive or reflect great responsibility or leadership roles. Also, it highlights periods when the candidate may have worked with or for well-recognized or highly reputable employers. In certain situations, this type of résumé should not be used. Specifically, it is inappropriate when the candidate has a rather sporadic job history, when continuity of employment or involvement is lacking, or when the applicant has a long list of rather short-lived positions. In addition, this type of résumé is not useful for those in the process of making a career change, or in situations where the work history is irrelevant to the position sought. Figure 11-1 contains an example of a (reverse) chronological résumé.

Thomas Moody, R.H.I.T., C.P.C.
1234 Sunnyside Dr.
Smalltown, FL 32851
Phone 352.421.1305 Email: tmoody43@anysite.com

Objective

To assist a hospital system in medical record compliance and in obtaining reimbursement optimally through proficiency in electronic claims procedures.

Employment History

March 2002 – present   **Medical Records Technician and Billing Representative**
                              Sunnyside Family Practice, Smalltown, FL

                              • Evaluate and ensure accuracy of patient medical records
                              • Submit electronic claims utilizing Medical Manager
                              • Train new employees in administrative tasks

April 1998 – March 2002   **Medical Billing Representative**
                              Medibill Solutions, Tampa, FL

                              • Utilized Medisoft program for claims submission
                              • Utilized ICD-9 and CPT-4 coding skills
                              • Assisted in office administration

May 1993 – April 1998   **Medical Administrative Assistant and Transcriptionist**
                              Janson Chiropractic and Wellness Center, West Town, VA

                              • Assisted with reception, patient check-in forms, and filing
                              • Transcribed office medical reports at 60 WPM
                              • Maintained office supply inventory

Summary of Qualifications/Credentials

Registered Health Information Technician   January 2000 – present
Certified Professional Coder   July 1999 – present
HIPAA course certification   May 1999 – present

Education

A.S. Degree   Health Information Technology   Myers College   May 1999
Diploma   Medical Office Assistant   FL Career Academy   May 2000

Figure 11-1. Example of a Chronological Résumé.

The Functional Résumé   The functional résumé can be thought of as a skills-based résumé. It accentuates the candidate's professional strengths, skills, and capabilities by showing where and how he or she has applied these in various positions or areas of specialty.

Those who lack any significant formal work history, perhaps young graduates seeking their first "real" job, should organize their capabilities and experiences in this format. Also, those who have been involved in various positions or functions in which professional skills and responsibilities were applied and those with no particular career path should organize their résumé in this way. Clear-cut and precise words and statements must be used to communicate these qualifications. The functional résumé should *not* be utilized when actual achievements gained or talents applied in past positions may be perceived as ambiguous.

Generally, the functional résumé emphasizes skills and qualifications to compensate for a relatively short or undeveloped work history. Figure 11-2 contains an example of a functional résumé.

Phoebe Turner, C.M.A.
1550 Callaway Dr. #202
Sandy Shores, SC 88921
Phone 881-412-9001 Email pturner@anysite.com

Summary of Qualifications
- AAMA Certified Medical Assistant - proficient in phlebotomy, injections, EKG, vitals, x-ray, patient education, medical billing, and front office procedures
- Leadership and supervisory skills
- Excellent time management in multitasking within fast-paced environment
- Efficient computer operation skills in Microsoft Word, Excel, and Access
- Typing speed 55 WPM

Experience
Medical Assisting
- Completed 300 externship hours - Oceanside Family Medicine, Sandy Shores, SC
- 150 hours front office/150 hours back office

Leadership/Supervising/Time Management
- Managed restaurant staff of 35 with high rates of customer satisfaction
- Supervised front desk staff of large law firm
- Served as Vice-President in homeowners association; participated with board members in making community improvements

Computer Performance
- Performed secretarial work within law firm office utilizing Microsoft Office suite programs, proving versatile for many computer tasks.
- Produced professional legal documents at 55 WPM, contributing to overall paperwork efficiency.

Employment History
Staff Manager	Oceanside Seafood Grill	April 1992 – May 1996
Legal Secretary	Martin, Bland, and Associates	August 1999 – March 2003

Education
A. S. Degree in Medical Assisting	Hillside Community College	May 2006
Office Administration Diploma	Technical Institute of Boca	October 1998

References available upon request.

Figure 11-2.   Example of a Functional Résumé.

The Combination Résumé   The combination résumé combines the objectives of both the chronological and functional résumé types into a hybrid form, usually by first specifying the candidate's qualifications, skills, and accomplishments and then showing the chronological work history. In this type of résumé, the candidate can showcase his or her best professional attributes and employment history. When both of these areas for any particular candidate will be impressive to an employer, this résumé format is advisable.

This format is beneficial when work history is varied, when externship or volunteer experience is to be included, and when changing career fields. It is helpful for demonstrating how a person has exercised the transferable skills he or she claims to possess.

Transferable skills are those skills that are useful, beneficial, and applicable to a wide range of other professional positions. Some examples include but are not limited to planning and implementing, managing, supervising, designing, coordinating, multitasking, assessing, training, utilizing computer skills, and presenting. In using these terms, it is important to clearly show what tasks these skills were used to accomplish. A combination résumé should *not* be used when even partially relevant work experience is lacking or when specific skills, qualifications, and achievements are not identifiable.

Examples of Transferable Skills

Human Relations–Focused Skills

- Listening
- Motivating
- Counseling
- Cooperating
- Establishing rapport
- Supporting

Planning, Organizing, and Management-Focused Skills

- Analyzing
- Solving
- Identifying
- Forecasting
- Initiating
- Decision making
- Delegating
- Promoting
- Coordinating

- Evaluating
- Implementing

Communication-Focused Skills

- Reporting
- Persuading
- Interviewing
- Negotiating
- Effectively writing and speaking
- Giving presentations
- Leading staff meetings

Professionalism/Work Ability–Focused Skills

- Managing time effectively
- Being punctual
- Demonstrating dependability
- Meeting set goals
- Meeting deadlines
- Organizing
- Cooperating
- Attending to details

Figure 11-3 contains an example of a combination résumé.

The Entry-Level Résumé   For students entering the allied health industry as a first profession (i.e., without prior work experience in any other industry), the résumé can be formatted to emphasize the skills and knowledge possessed despite this lack of experience. In this type of résumé, it is especially important to document the externship experience. Other key details to include in this type of résumé are technical skills related to your chosen allied health specialty, certifications you have obtained as a result of your training, and any part-time, full-time, or volunteer positions you have held. Even if you perceive this bit of experience as useless in your pursuit of professional work, you should still document the experience as it shows that you were actively participating in the workforce (rather than sitting at home watching TV!). Overall, this résumé format provides details of the recent training you have completed and shows that you are focused on building a successful career from this starting point.

When presenting this type of résumé to prospective employers, keep in mind that your interviews become even more important. In light of less experience, interviewers may be more critical of your responses and interview etiquette than

John Smith, C.Ph.T.
1221 33rd Street North
Perry, FL 54321
508-513-9800 / jsmith79@anysite.com

Objective
To contribute to hospital pharmacy productivity while advancing in technical skills and
pharmacy staff teamwork and leadership.

Relevant Skills
- Professional competency in pharmacy technology – C.Ph.T.
- Retail pharmacy technical and customer service skills for 2+ years
- Small business management (inventory, accounting and financial management)
  for 7+ years
- Computer skills (Windows and MacIntosh programs) utilized in all positions held
  using spreadsheet, database, and word processing applications

Experience
8/2005 – present: Pharmacy Technician; XYZ Pharmacy, Perry, FL
    Maintained inventory, verified customer insurance, filled prescriptions, observed
    quality control procedures, helped ensure superior customer service.

6/1997 – 9/2004: Manager; ABC Shipping, Tallahassee, FL
    Managed finances, inventory, and operations of small shipping company;
    maintained increasing revenues and profits steadily each year; ensured
    customer retention through customer satisfaction.

7/1993 – 5/1997: Customer Service Representative, TalkCom Telephone Service Co.,
    Atlanta, GA. Addressed customer inquiries and complaints; collaborated with
    division management to help resolve customer issues; presented telephone
    package options to interested customers.

Education
1995   A.A. degree in Business Management   Southern Community College
2005   A.S. degree in Pharmacy Technology   Health Sciences Technical Institute

Figure 11-3.   An Example of a Combination Résumé

those of a candidate possessing five or more successful years of professional
experience. Figure 11-4 contains an example of a suitable entry-level résumé.

Including Allied Health Information in the Résumé

Regardless of the type of résumé used, the allied health candidate should also include some very specific and relevant pieces of information. First, include the title
of the credential earned in the area of specialization. Some examples are the Certified or Registered Medical Assistant (CMA or RMA), Registered Health Information Technician (RHIT), Certified Professional Coder (CPC), Certified Pharmacy
Technician (CPhT), and so on. This will clearly demonstrate competency.

Portia Edwards
2000 Pine Arbor Dr
Orlando, FL 55555
Cell: 777-555-3333 Email: pedwards43@anysite.com

Objective
To obtain a position as a Medical Assistant in a successful organization where my skills and education can be utilized.

Education
Florida Technical College, Orlando FL   Jan 2008
Associate of Science, Medical Assisting   GPA 3.58

Certifications
Certified Medical Assistant
CPR Certified

Skills
- Bilingual (Spanish)
- Microsoft Word, Excel, PowerPoint
- Medisoft
- Vital signs
- EKG's
- Phlebotomy
- Medication administration / injections
- Collection and processing of laboratory specimens
- Phoning/faxing in prescription refills to pharmacy
- Faxing referral information
- Scheduling appointments
- Chart documentation
- Filing/pulling medical charts

Experience

Oct 2007 – Jan 2008 Medical Assistant Extern	Premcare Family Medical Center 300 hrs; Front and Back Office	Orlando, FL
Aug 2006 – Present Hostess/Waitress	Donatos Pizza	Orlando, FL
Apr 2005 – Jun 2005 Baker/Cashier	Acme Markets	Middlesex, NJ
Aug 2003 – Aug 2004 Assistant Manager	Brooklyn Bakery	Middlesex, NJ

References Available Upon Request

Figure 11-4 Example of an Entry-Level Résumé.
Source: Contributed by Veena Garib, MBA, Career Services Director, Technical/Career College.

Recent graduates with only externship experience in the field should include technical and clinical skills within the field in which employment is sought. Any other supportive certifications and coursework should be listed, such as BLS, CPR, and First Aid certification, HIPAA certification, phlebotomy certification,

EKG/ECG certification, and the like. Inclusion of all competency areas is of special importance when applying for jobs in allied health.

Recommendations for Résumé Formatting and Writing

The overall look and clarity of the résumé you provide will influence how you are perceived professionally by anyone who screens résumés and interviewers. When numerous résumés are collected by the employer, it is likely that only the best applicants (according to what is seen on the résumé) will be contacted for an interview.

Thus, you should view your résumé as your one and only application for an interview. If the résumé is sloppy, disorganized, or unappealing for any reason, the résumé screener may send it to the shredder.

Your goal should be to create an attractive, easy-to-follow, and organized résumé with wording that makes a bold impression concerning your skills, experience, education, and so on. The following lists highlight some aspects of formatting and writing to which you should adhere as you develop the "look" and "sound" of your résumé.

Appropriate Formatting

- The résumé must be pleasing to the eye and attractive to the reader.
- The résumé must be clear and easy to follow, which is accomplished with appropriate spacing, indentations, headings, and punctuation. It should not contain lengthy, detailed paragraphs that make the page look too wordy. Brief, bulleted lists showing highlights under each heading are effective and create an organized look.
- The font used for the résumé should be kept simple, with font size kept in the average range of 10 to 14 points. The use of fancy or stylish graphics and shading is unnecessary for allied health résumés. *Never* submit a handwritten résumé to an employer.
- The résumé should be printed on very light-colored or white, good-quality paper for in-person distribution.
- The design of the résumé should grab the reader's attention and draw it to the most important aspects the résumé is intended to highlight.

Appropriate Writing

- Use relevant power words from your profession and action verbs to clearly identify your capabilities and experiences.
- Be sure that your grammar and spelling are impeccable. If an employer views a résumé with even a very few or very minor errors of this nature, he or she will likely disregard the represented candidate.
- Use an appropriate, professional-looking e-mail address within the contact information area of the résumé. E-mail addresses using silly or vulgar words,

slang terms, or inappropriate implications will not amuse the résumé reader or potential employer and may actually cause them to discard your résumé.

- If your experience is irrelevant to the work you seek, list the appropriate transferable skills (such as those listed previously in this chapter) that link your professional attributes to your new area of expertise.
- Through your written expression of previous experiences and relevant skills or qualifications, create a professional image that matches the prestige and salary you desire.
- Prioritize according to significance the information that falls under each heading or position title.
- Sell the benefits of your skills and qualifications by including how your skills are of benefit to the potential employer.

Finalizing the Résumé

Once you have completed your résumé, ask a few other individuals, including the career resource professionals at your school, to critique the wording and format. Then make the appropriate adjustments. Always save an electronic copy on the hard drive of your personal computer and on an external disk. Keep a professional binder, organizer, or folder handy with several copies of your résumé on good quality paper.

The Cover Letter

Your overall goal for submitting a cover letter with your résumé is to stir up an employer's interest in you as a possible candidate for an open position, while adding a slight personal touch. Any cover letter for an allied health position should reflect that you have some experience, at least an externship, as well as some formal education and training in the field you are pursuing. More important, though, you must strive to sell yourself by "advertising" what you are able to do for the employer.

For example, you should briefly explain how your skills can contribute to the efficiency of the facility, hospital, pharmacy, or office, as well as how your experience and accomplishments in past positions will benefit this employer. Do not be too lengthy in making your points, though. The reader will want to move quickly through your brief and concise cover letter.

The tone of the cover letter should be conversational. Avoid using what you think might be big and impressive words, as letters with too much of this hyped-up terminology and pretentious words or phrases are often quite unattractive to the reader. Be yourself, but use proper wording, spelling, and punctuation, with the personal touch of thought and creativity. An effective and impressive way to add this personal touch is to briefly describe how you can apply your personal or professional experience to help the company meet or exceed its goals. Try to be specific in aligning your abilities with the company's goals, which can be customer service oriented, production oriented, growth oriented, or efficiency oriented, among other types of business goals. Mentioning this in the cover letter will demonstrate that you have put thought into this company even prior to an interview and will highlight a portion of your personal qualifications for the position, which the potential employer will find quite impressive.

Always keep an electronic copy of your cover letter accessible so that you can alter the name and company/organization to which the letter is directed. You also can easily modify the letter as necessary when applying to several different employers. Figure 11-5 provides an example of a cover letter.

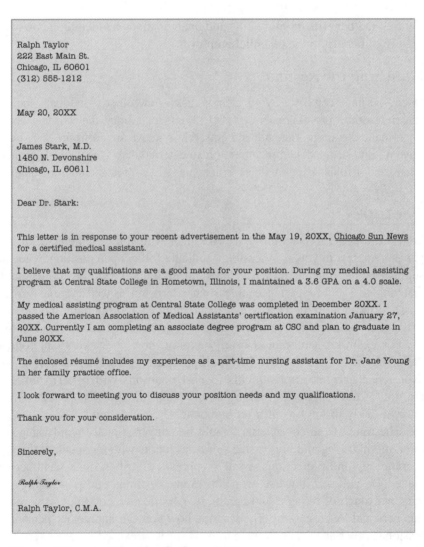

Ralph Taylor
222 East Main St.
Chicago, IL 60601
(312) 555-1212

May 20, 20XX

James Stark, M.D.
1450 N. Devonshire
Chicago, IL 60611

Dear Dr. Stark:

This letter is in response to your recent advertisement in the May 19, 20XX, <u>Chicago Sun News</u> for a certified medical assistant.

I believe that my qualifications are a good match for your position. During my medical assisting program at Central State College in Hometown, Illinois, I maintained a 3.6 GPA on a 4.0 scale.

My medical assisting program at Central State College was completed in December 20XX. I passed the American Association of Medical Assistants' certification examination January 27, 20XX. Currently I am completing an associate degree program at CSC and plan to graduate in June 20XX.

The enclosed résumé includes my experience as a part-time nursing assistant for Dr. Jane Young in her family practice office.

I look forward to meeting you to discuss your position needs and my qualifications.

Thank you for your consideration.

Sincerely,

Ralph Taylor

Ralph Taylor, C.M.A.

Figure 11-5.   An Example of a Cover Letter.

The Waiting Period

The waiting period refers to the time between submitting your résumés in response to job postings and receiving a response to your expressed interest. You have a few issues to consider during this time.

One very important fact is that an employer may contact you, most likely by phone, at any time. In the current age of multifunctional cell phones, voice-mails that play musical messages, music clips that play for callers while they await call pickup, and the like, many young adults and others are fascinated by this technology and subscribe to these services. While these are fun and amusing products of our time, they are *not in the least* fun *or* amusing to potential employers who are contacting you for a professional interview. What do you suppose an employer would think or do when greeted by a recording that plays a clip from a questionable rap song? Suppose the voice-mail message sounds something like "Yeah, hey, I ain't here now; leave a message," with audible TV and other background sounds muffling the entire message. How would this caller respond as a potential employer of a candidate who offered such a message? A highly likely response might be to hang up the phone and move on to the next candidate. Therefore, it is very important for your professional image during this job search phase to come across as "normal," mature, and professional to anyone who contacts you. A simple message—such as "Hello, you have reached the voice mail of John Doe. Please leave a message. I will return your call as soon as possible. Thanks."—will be much more acceptable and respectable.

The next most popular form of communication from a potential employer is e-mail. The first and foremost issue with using e-mail as an available line of professional contact with potential employers is to offer a decent, professional-sounding e-mail address with your contact information, as briefly mentioned already in the section on résumé writing. Creative, amusing, and even vulgar language references are common today in many people's personal e-mail addresses, but you must avoid these if you are hoping to be selected for an interview. If you currently use a not-so-professional e-mail address, sign up under a respectable name for one that you can use for professional correspondence throughout your life. For example, a first initial and last name or some variation of your name and a meaningful number would be perfectly appropriate.

Examples of Unprofessional E-mail Addresses
- babygotback@somedomain.com
- chick4you@somedomain.com
- foreverhigh@somedomain.com

Such e-mail addresses are inappropriate because they all have vulgar intention built into them. While this may be fun for strictly social contacts, such addresses must *not* be used for professional contacts.

Examples of Professional E-mail Addresses

- kjcharles@somedomain.com
- becky43@somedomain.com
- jenna_bosworth@somedomain.com

Basic, straightforward, and unquestionable in nature, such e-mail addresses are acceptable and expected of employers seeking allied health professionals.

Another area to focus on during the waiting period is using your time to research the companies or practices to which you have submitted your application/résumé. The best and most convenient resource is the Web site, if one is maintained by the employer. (Small doctor's offices are less likely to have a Web site available than are larger organizations, such as hospitals, large health care groups or chains, insurance or managed care organizations, and pharmacies.) If a Web site is unavailable, phone or stop by the office or facility and ask if a brochure or some type of informative literature about the practice or organization is available. When taking this action on the premises, be sure to obtain a business card. Doing this during your waiting period will ensure that you are prepared for an interview, can speak intelligently concerning the respective organizations, and can ask meaningful or insightful questions when prompted during the interview. This indefinite time of waiting should not be wasted. Use it to your advantage.

The Interview

You will make your real first impression on a potential employer at the interview—and it's important that it be a good one. You should be mindful of your attire, as well as your etiquette, when preparing for the interview.

Dressing for the Interview

Professional attire and an overall professional appearance are necessary for a successful interview. As mentioned in Chapter 3, when attending an externship interview it may be appropriate to wear the scrubs that are normally considered your school uniform. This is not the case when interviewing for a job beyond the externship. A business suit is appropriate for such an interview.

Suits for interviews should be dark or neutral in color, well coordinated, and worn with appropriate dress shoes. Bright-colored suits or those with dramatic designs or prints should not be worn. Shoes should be neat, new in appearance, clean, and conservative in style.

Plan your interview attire so that you are sure all pieces are clean and pressed before the big day. Do not wear perfume on the day of the interview. Jewelry should be conservative, if worn at all: neat and moderate, not bold, big, or high-fashion. Remove jewelry or piercings beyond the ear lobe (e.g., upper ear, nose, eyebrow, and tongue piercings). Hair should be clean and styled neatly; avoid a high-fashion or dramatic hair design for the interview. Keep in mind that outrageously colorful highlights or hair color such as pink, blue, or green will automatically tell the interviewer not to take you seriously. Candidates with visible tattoos and untraditional piercings may send this message as well. Be sure to carry a professional-looking binder or folder containing additional copies of your résumé and cover letter.

Etiquette for the Interview

It is important to make the best impression possible during your interview. The following list highlights the various areas of interview etiquette that must be heeded to meet the expected and appropriate performance:

- Make a mental note of the name of your interviewer(s) so that you can offer thanks by name at the conclusion of your interview.
- Your efforts in making the best impression begin at the moment you arrive on the employer's property and continue to the moment you leave. If you drive to the property, do not enter or exit the parking area with loud music or bass vibrating. Everyone near a window will look to see who is responsible.
- Cell phones should be off and out of sight from the time of your arrival until you leave the premises, including while you are waiting to begin the interview.
- Arrive approximately ten minutes early. This will allow the employer and staff to notice before the interview begins that you are punctual . It also will provide time in case you are requested to complete forms or an application prior to meeting with the interviewer(s).
- Greet the interviewer with a pleasant smile and a firm handshake.
- Do not let your mind wander during the interview, even if the interviewer decides to give you a ten-minute detailed speech about the organization. Pay attention so that you can think of good, quality questions to ask the interviewer when appropriate.
- Maintain eye contact. Do not stare into space or look around, especially at your watch or the clock, while engaged in the conversation.
- Sit upright with good posture. Do not slouch or lean on your elbows.
- Answer the question asked. Do not extrapolate, bringing other insight or answers to questions that were not asked. Some questions will require simple, straightforward responses, and some will require explanations and examples.
- Use good manners, saying "Please," "Thank-you," "Excuse me," and so on.
- Avoid filler words that make you sound uncertain of what you are trying to say, such as "uh," "like," "you know." Keep your language simple. Do not try to use big words that are unnatural in conversation. Use technical terms only if the question asked requires you to use them to answer appropriately.

- Express confidence and competence throughout the interview, but do not brag or act haughtily.

At the end of the interview, thank the interviewer(s) (by name) and end with a firm handshake.

The Thank-You Letter

The appropriate time to send a thank-you letter to the person(s) who conducted the interview is within twenty-four hours of an interview. This letter should first thank those to whom it is addressed for taking time to meet with you, to discuss more about their organization and its needs, and to discuss your qualifications. Mention some aspect of the company or its needs that were discussed with you during the interview, and reiterate how that aligns with your interest, capabilities, and professional goals. If you would like the interviewers to know something relevant that was not mentioned in the interview, briefly mention it, as long as it ties into your statements and demonstrates a solid professional match between the organization and you. Before closing the letter, restate your appreciation for being considered for the position. With a thoughtful thank-you letter, you will add to any good impression you made. Figure 11-6 provides an example of a thank-you letter.

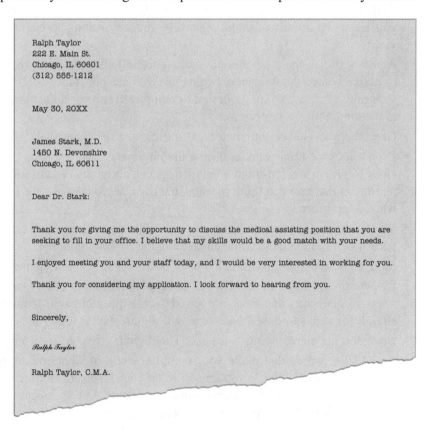

Ralph Taylor
222 E. Main St.
Chicago, IL 60601
(312) 555-1212

May 30, 20XX

James Stark, M.D.
1450 N. Devonshire
Chicago, IL 60611

Dear Dr. Stark:

Thank you for giving me the opportunity to discuss the medical assisting position that you are seeking to fill in your office. I believe that my skills would be a good match with your needs.

I enjoyed meeting you and your staff today, and I would be very interested in working for you.

Thank you for considering my application. I look forward to hearing from you.

Sincerely,

Ralph Taylor

Ralph Taylor, C.M.A.

Figure 11-6.   An Example of a Thank-You Letter.

HIGHLIGHT: Tips from Professionals

"Remember these few tips to have a good interview and make a good impression:

- Plan to be early. It not only makes a good impression, but it will save you if an unexpected obstacle comes up the day of the interview.
- Dress professionally. Depending on your profession, this could mean wearing different clothes than you would on the job. For example, don't wear scrubs for a job interview.
- Bring your résumé. Even if you have already provided the employer with a copy of your résumé, bring a hard copy with you to the interview.
- Answer questions thoroughly, but don't ramble. And remember that simple 'yes' and 'no' answers are too brief.
- Make eye contact. Making eye contact with the interviewer shows that you are confident and have an interest in the job and the person conducting the interview.
- After the interview, thank the interviewer for his or her time. A nice extra step would be to send a thank-you note or e-mail. It could make the difference if the decision to be made (regarding hiring you) is tough."

Kevin A. Lenhart,
MHS, Health Services Director, County Sheriff's Office

CONCLUSION

As you have now determined, searching for employment is almost a full-time job in itself. You can optimize your opportunities by first becoming familiar with your local job market and resources for scouting open positions in your allied health specialty. Carefully formulating your résumé to reflect the best possible professional image of yourself is of primary importance since in most cases your résumé is the first representation of you that employers will see. An impressive cover letter expresses your interests in the employers to whom you are submitting your application, while demonstrating your compatibility for the position and your abilities that will meet the employer's needs.

The interview is your time to shine. Prepare to make your best impression and to demonstrate confidence. Follow up the interview with a brief but meaningful thank-you letter to show your appreciation for the interview opportunity and to reiterate your interest in the available position.

Self-Prep Questions

In addition to considering the following questions as you prepare for your job search, review the Self-Prep Questions in Chapter 3.

1. List your most accessible resources for beginning your job search.

_____

_____

_____

_____

_____

_____

_____

_____

_____

_____

_____

2. Which type of résumé is most effective for you personally, considering your work history, education, externship/internships, volunteer activity, and so on? Why?

_____

_____

_____

_____

_____

_____

_____

_____

_____

_____

3. New allied health graduates come from diverse employment and educational backgrounds. List at least three transferable skills from your work history or other activities that will be useful to mention on your résumé and during interview(s).

_____

_____

_____

_____

_____

_____

_____

_____

_____

4. List a few terms that you could choose from for briefly but concisely and effectively "selling yourself" in your cover letter. Be sure that these are supported by your actual accomplishments, and relate them to how they will likely assist the employer in achieving company goals.

_____

_____

_____

_____

_____

_____

_____

_____

_____

Role-Play Scenario

This scenario requires two individuals. One individual is an interviewer, and the other is a candidate for employment at an organization relevant to the candidate's allied health specialty. The group or class participating in this should plan the activity in advance so that arriving to the interview on time, appropriately and professionally dressed, and with a résumé can be practiced. Interviewers should gather appropriate interview questions from their school's career resource staff, from their instructors, or from researching interview questions on the Internet or other sources. Interviews should be approximately ten minutes long (or more) for this activity.

1. In what ways has the candidate given a good first impression?

_____

_____

_____

_____

_____

_____

_____

_____

_____

_____

2. In what areas could the candidate improve to give a better impression?

_____

_____

_____

_____

_____

_____

_____

_____

_____

3. Based on the etiquette, appearance, and communication tactics employed by the candidate during the interview, what is your perception about his or her level of professionalism and ability to perform well in the prospective job?

_____

_____

_____

_____

_____

_____

_____

_____

_____

_____

✓ Readiness Checklist

_____ I understand that to be successful in the job search, I must be proactive in working through each step of the process.

_____ I know which local resources are most accessible and most valuable to me in beginning my job search.

_____ I understand the importance of my résumé in capturing and holding the attention of potential employers.

_____ I understand the general differences among chronological, functional, combination, and entry-level résumés.

_____ I know which résumé format is most suitable for my use.

_____ I understand the meaning of "transferable skills."

_____ I realize the importance of appropriate formatting and writing for my résumé.

_____ I have thought of ways to "sell myself" in my cover letter by emphasizing how I can help my potential employer(s) accomplish organizational goals, based on my own achievements and experiences.

_____ I understand the importance of utilizing normal voice-mail messages during the waiting period, when I could be receiving responses from potential employers.

_____ During the waiting period, I realize that I should spend time wisely by researching those employers to whom I have applied, so that I am well prepared for an interview at any time.

_____ I understand the appropriate style of dress required for an interview.

_____ I understand the various manners expected and those not to exhibit during an interview.

_____ I understand that within twenty-four hours of any interview, I should prove my professionalism by sending the interviewer an appropriately written thank-you letter.

_____ I have saved or will save a copy of my résumé in electronic format so that I can easily update it when appropriate.

_____ I am prepared to succeed in the launch of my allied health career!

appendix

Selected Allied-Health Certification and Credentialing Resources

American Academy of Professional Coders (AAPC)

Credentials Awarded: CPC (Certified Professional Coder)
CPC-H (Certified Professional Coder–Hospital)
CPC-P (Certified Professional Coder–Payer)
And more.
On the Internet: www.aapc.com

The American Association of Medical Assistants (AAMA)

Credential Awarded: CMA (AAMA) (Certified Medical Assistant)
On the Internet: www.aama-ntl.org

American Dental Assistants Association (ADAA)

Professional organization in alliance with DANB
On the Internet: www.dentalassistant.org

American Health Information Management Association (AHIMA)

Credentials awarded: RHIT (Registered Health Information Technician)
RHIA (Registered Health Information Administrator)
On the Internet: www.ahima.org

American Medical Technologists (AMT)

Credentials Awarded: RMA (Registered Medical Assistant)
RPT (Registered Phlebotomy Technician)
RDA (Registered Dental Assistant)
CMAS (Certified Medical Administrative Specialist)

MT (Medical Technologist)
And more.
On the Internet: www.amt1.com

Association of Surgical Technologists (AST)

Professional Organization
On the Internet: www.ast.org

Dental Assisting National Board, Inc. (DANB)

Credentials awarded: CDA (Certified Dental Assistant)
COA (Certified Orthodontic Assistant)
CDPMA (Certified Dental Practice Management Administrator)
On the Internet: www.dentalassisting.com

National Board of Surgical Technology and Surgical Assisting (NBSTSA)

Credential Awarded: CST (Certified Surgical Technologist)
CFA (Certified First Assistant)
On the Internet: www.nbstsa.org

National Center for Competency Testing (NCCT)

Credentials Awarded: NCMA (National Certified Medical Assistant)
NCMOA (National Certified Medical Office Assistant)
NCET (National Certified ECG Technician)
NCPT (National Certified Phlebotomy Technician)
NCPhT (National Certified Pharmacy Technician)
NCICS (National Certified Insurance and Coding Specialist)
And more.
On the Internet: www.ncctinc.com

Pharmacy Technician Certification Board (PTCB)

Credential Awarded: CPhT (Certified Pharmacy Technician)
On the Internet: www.ptcb.org

Journal

Index